Cleft Lip and Palate

Cleft Lip and Palate
a team approach

Edited by
E.H. Albery, I.S. Hathorn and R.W. Pigott
Frenchay Hospital, Bristol

WRIGHT
Bristol
1986

Published by
John Wright & Sons Ltd, Techno House, Redcliffe Way, Bristol BS1 6NX

British Library Cataloguing in Publication Data

Cleft lip and palate: a team approach.
  1. Orthodontics   2. Harelip — Therapy
  3. Cleft palate — Therapy
  I. Albery, E.H.   II. Hathorn, I.S.
  III. Pigott, R.W.
  617′.522   RK527

ISBN 0 7236 0700 1

Printed in Great Britain by
Adlard & Son Ltd, Dorking, Surrey

Preface

Fifteen thousand children are born each year in the United Kingdom with clefts of the lip and palate. About half of these will continue to need the help of cleft palate teams until they have finished growing and even beyond. Therefore about 15 000 patients will be in need of advice at any time. Apart from cleft palate team members, patients will often seek advice from many other sources, for example from their general practitioner, dentist or health visitor. The book provides an introduction to all major aspects of cleft lip and palate, from embryology and anatomy, surgery, dental care and orthodontics, and speech and hearing to feeding, genetic counselling and family support. Illustrations are shown throughout many chapters. Although written from one centre, particular care has been exercised to avoid a dogmatic approach to a subject about which there are conflicting views.

This book is intended to provide sufficient information to enable those who are professionally involved to give answers to their patients' questions. It has also been written with the intention that it could be read by parents who would like to understand some of the thinking behind the management of their child's deformity.

Finally, it will provide an introduction to the subject for students of medicine, dentistry, speech therapy and nursing.

E.H.A.
R.W.P.
I.H.

Contributors

E.H. Albery BSc, LCST
Speech Therapist, Frenchay Hospital, Bristol

B.K.B. Berkovitz MSc, BDS, PhD, LDS, RCS
Anatomy Department, University of Bristol

I.S. Hathorn BDS, FDS, DOrth, RCS
Consultant Orthodontist, Frenchay Hospital and Dental Hospital, Bristol

A.R. Maw MB, FRCS
Consultant Otolaryngologist, Bristol Royal Infirmary and Royal Hospital for Sick Children, Bristol

J. Osborne MD, MRCP
Consultant Paediatrician, Royal United Hospital, Bath

G. Pell MB, BS, BDS, FDS, RCS, MRCS, LRCP
Consultant Oral Surgeon, Frenchay Hospital, Bristol

R.W. Pigott BA, MB, BCh, BAO, FRCS, FRCSI
Consultant Plastic Surgeon, Frenchay Hospital, Bristol

J.M. Smith BSc(Econ.), CQSW
Avon Social Services Department

Contents

Chapter 1

Embryology

B.K.B. Berkovitz

Facial development becomes evident during the fourth week after fertilization, with the appearance of five prominences or swellings around a shallow depression representing the stomodeum (primitive oral cavity) (*Fig.* 1.1). Such swellings are traditionally termed 'facial processes'. The central swelling above the stomodeum is the frontonasal process. Situated laterally and below the stomodeum are the two mandibular processes, whilst at the corners of the stomodeum are the maxillary processes. The frontonasal process contributes to the development of the nose (and possibly upper lip), the mandibular processes to the development of the lower jaw and lip and the maxillary processes to the upper jaw and lip. The facial processes result from accumulations of mesenchymal cells beneath the surface epithelium. These mesenchymal cells are of neural crest (ectomesenchymal) origin, having migrated from the site of the developing neural tube into the head region where they make a significant contribution to the development of many oro-facial structures (e.g. nerves, teeth, bones, oral mucosa). The cells produce the elevations of the branchial arches from the first of which arise the mandibular and maxillary facial processes. Initially, the stomodeum (lined by ectoderm) is separated posteriorly from the pharynx (lined by endoderm) by a bilaminar (ectodermal/endodermal) membrane termed the 'buccopharyngeal' membrane. However, this membrane degenerates by the end of the fourth week establishing continuity between the oral cavity and pharynx (*Fig.* 1.2).

DEVELOPMENT OF NASAL CAVITIES AND PALATE

Two zones of epithelium on the frontonasal process become delineated to form the nasal placodes (*Fig.* 1.1). These placodes will eventually form the specialized olfactory epithelium found in the roof of the nasal cavity. During

1

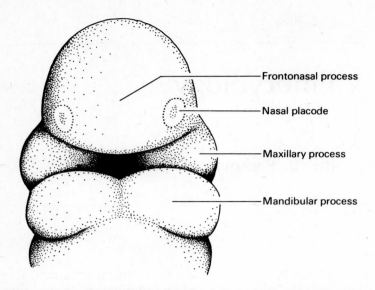

Fig. 1.1. Frontal aspect of face during fourth week of development.

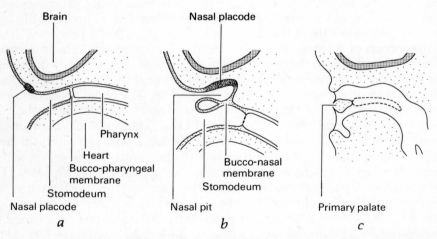

Fig. 1.2. Sagittal sections of head showing development of primary nasal cavities. (*a*) 4 weeks; (*b*) 5 weeks; (*c*) 6 weeks.

the fifth week, each nasal placode sinks into the underlying mesenchyme and lies in the roof of an epithelial-lined invagination termed a 'nasal pit' (*Fig.* 1.2). The margins of each nasal pit become enlarged both laterally and medially as a result of the accumulation of underlying mesenchymal cells to form lateral and medial nasal processes (*Fig.* 1.3). The midline region incorporating the medial nasal processes is sometimes referred to as the globular process.

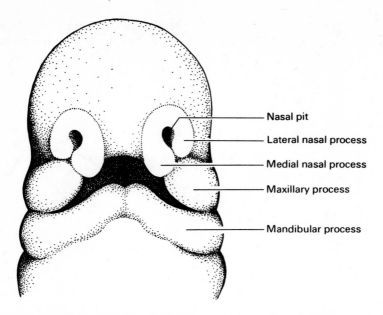

Nasal pit

Lateral nasal process

Medial nasal process

Maxillary process

Mandibular process

Fig. 1.3. Frontal aspect of face during fifth week of development.

The nasal pits extend deeper into the underlying mesenchyme, gradually approaching the epithelium lining the roof of the stomodeum. Eventually, only an epithelial membrane, the bucconasal membrane, separates the oral and nasal cavities. Breakdown of this membrane at the end of the fifth week establishes continuity between oral and nasal cavities (*Fig.* 1.2). The nasal cavities so far described are termed the 'primary nasal cavities'. The tissue of the frontonasal process in the midline which separates the two primary nasal cavities from each other is termed the 'primary nasal septum'; that which separates the primary nasal cavities from the primary oral cavity is termed the 'primary palate'. The reason for the use of the adjective 'primary' in these situations can be deduced with reference to *Figs* 1.2 and 1.4. Compared to the definitive nasal cavities, the nasal cavities so far described only extend back to the approximate level of the future incisive foramen. It is only with further extension backwards of the palate (secondary palate) and nasal septum (secondary nasal septum) that the common oro-nasal cavity is divided into oral and nasal chambers and the full extent of the definitive nasal cavities becomes evident.

The secondary palate becomes apparent during the sixth week of development. Palatal shelves grow horizontally from each maxillary process into the common oro-nasal cavity lying behind the primary palate (*Fig.* 1.4). Because of the presence of the developing tongue which occupies a considerable part of the oro-nasal cavity, the palatal shelves are deflected downwards and, during the seventh week, can be seen lying vertically (*Fig.* 1.5). During the eighth week, two crucial events occur, the mechanisms of which are poorly understood. First, the tongue appears to move, or is displaced, from its position between the palatal shelves, and no longer forms

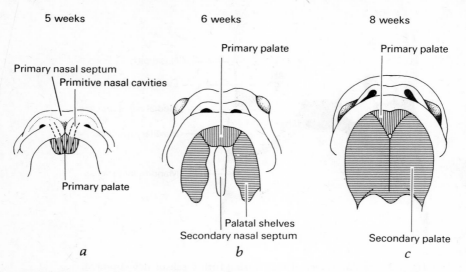

Fig. 1.4. Development of the palate. (*a*) 5 weeks; (*b*) 6 weeks; (*c*) 8 weeks.

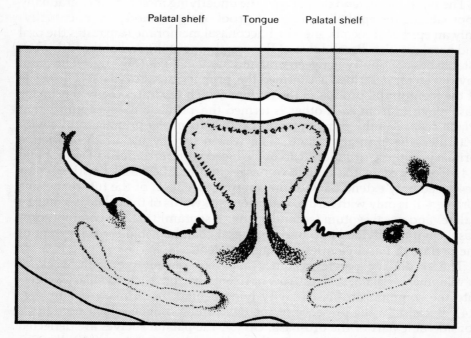

Fig. 1.5. Coronal section through a developing decalcified head during the seventh week of development.

a physical barrier between them. Second, the palatal shelves change from a vertical to a horizontal disposition, contacting each other in the midline and contacting the primary palate anteriorly (*Figs* 1.4 and 1.6). In this way, the common oro-nasal cavity is divided into separate oral and nasal cavities continuous with the respective primary cavities anteriorly.

Palatal shelf elevation probably occurs rapidly if the human situation is in any way comparable to that seen in rodents where a change from the vertical to the horizontal position can occur literally in seconds. The palatal shelves initially meet and fuse about one-third of the way back. Fusion then spreads both forwards and backwards. An increase in the adhesive properties of the free surfaces of the shelves where they contact may occur around the time of fusion.

In addition to the secondary palate, a secondary nasal septum develops behind the primary nasal septum from the roof of the oro-nasal cavity. It eventually fuses in the midline with the elevated palatal shelves, dividing the common nasal cavity into right and left chambers (*Figs* 1.4 and 1.6).

Fusion between the palatal shelves, nasal septum and primary palate results in mesenchymal continuity between the tissues. This fusion is

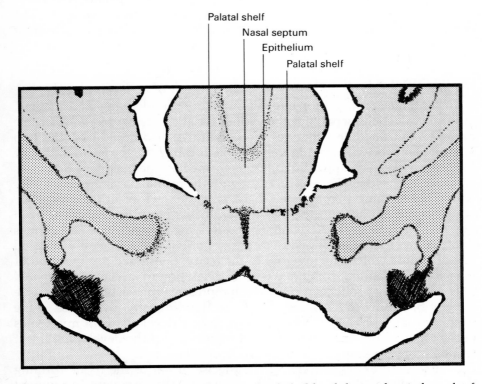

Fig. 1.6. Coronal section through developing decalcified head during the ninth week of development.

achieved by the removal of epithelium which initially separates the different regions (*Fig.* 1.6). This could occur by two separate processes:

1. By the flattening out of grooves due to movement of underlying mesenchyme.
2. By degeneration and subsequent removal of epithelium.

In this context, it is generally stated that when the palatal shelves contact each other in the midline, the intervening epithelium undergoes programmed cell death. Whether such degeneration is an inbuilt property of the palatal epithelial cells or is in any way influenced by the underlying mesenchyme awaits clarification. Fusion of the palate commences in the eighth week, and is complete by about the twelfth week of development. In the adult, the site at which the three palatal components meet is represented by the incisive papilla which overlies the incisive canal. Ossification occurs intramembranously from four centres in the anterior two-thirds of the palate destined to form the hard palate. The posterior one-third of the palate behind the nasal septum remains unossified as the soft palate. It is invaded by muscles originating from the branchial arches. These are the tensor palati from the first arch and the levator palati, palatoglossus, palatopharyngeus and musculus uvula, all probably from the fourth branchial arch. The different embryological origins of the muscles help explain their different nerve supply.

DEVELOPMENT OF THE FACE

With continued proliferation and migration of the underlying mesenchyme, the grooves initially separating the various facial processes gradually become flattened out and the processes merge with each other. Thus, the two mandibular processes meet in the midline, forming the lower boundary of the oral cavity. The upper boundary is formed by the maxillary processes growing in on either side and merging with the medial nasal processes (*Fig.* 1.3). This merging is complete by the seventh week of development.

A sheet of epithelium, the primary epithelial band, grows down from the surface of the oral cavity into the underlying mesenchyme and divides into two, a labially positioned vestibular lamina and a lingually situated dental lamina which will give rise to the teeth. Continued proliferation of the vestibular lamina, combined with degeneration of its centrally situated cells, eventually produces a cleft which represents the vestibule, the tissue labially becoming the lips and cheek and that lingually giving rise to the teeth and jaws (*Fig.* 1.7). The lip musculature develops from myotomes in the second branchial arch and as it migrates into the developing lips it retains its nerve supply (facial nerve) from this arch.

Controversy exists concerning the precise origin of the tissue forming the medial third of the upper lip. One view holds that, as might be apparent from *Fig.* 1.3, the middle third is derived from the medial nasal processes, whilst the lateral thirds are formed from the two maxillary processes. An

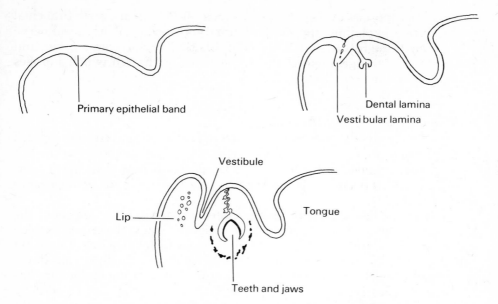

Fig. 1.7. Development of vestibule (cheek furrow).

alternative view is that the two maxillary processes overgrow the medial nasal processes and meet in the midline, thereby contributing all the tissue of the upper lip. This view is based upon an appreciation of the innervation of the upper lip which is entirely from the maxillary nerve which innervates tissue derived embryologically from the maxillary process (tissue derived from the frontonasal process being supplied by the ophthalmic nerve).

DEVELOPMENT OF TONGUE

The tongue develops from the floor of the pharynx. The anterior two-thirds arises from the first branchial arch (hence its general sensory supply from the lingual nerve), the posterior one-third chiefly from the third branchial arch but with a contribution from the fourth (hence its general sensory supply from the glossopharyngeal nerve with an additional component from the vagus nerve). The muscles of the tongue migrate into it from their initial position in the occipital region, carrying their innervation from the hypoglossal nerve with them.

DEVELOPMENT OF LARYNX

The thyroid cartilage develops from the fourth branchial arch, whilst the cricoid, arytenoid, corniculate and cuneiform cartilages probably develop from the sixth branchial arch. The epiglottis develops from the fourth arch.

The intrinsic muscles of the larynx arise from the fourth and sixth branchial arches, hence explaining their innervation by the external laryngeal nerve (the nerve of the fourth arch which supplies the cricothyroid muscle) and the recurrent laryngeal nerve (the nerve of the sixth arch which supplies all the remaining muscles).

CLEFTS OF LIP AND PALATE

One particular developmental defect which has a profound effect on speech is cleft formation. Once knowledge of the normal development of the lips and palate is obtained, it becomes easier to appreciate how clefts may occur. Cleft lip and cleft palate are thought to have a polygenic mode of inheritance (*see* Chapter 11).

Clefts of the lips appear to be associated primarily with defects of the mesenchyme which fails to proliferate or migrate. Thus, the grooves which early on in development demarcate the various facial swellings fail to fill out normally. The tissue remaining in these regions eventually breaks down with resulting cleft formation. It is not known whether the epithelium has more than a passive role to play in the aetiology of cleft lip. Depending upon the extent of the defect, the degree of clefting may vary from slight grooving to a complete cleft of the lip. If the defect lies between the maxillary and medial nasal processes, the cleft is situated to one side of the upper lip (either unilaterally or bilaterally). More rarely, defects between the medial nasal processes or between the mandibular processes give rise to median clefts.

Cleft palate may result from conditions which interfere with normal growth, elevation, adherence and fusion of the secondary palatal shelves, and/or which interfere with fusion between primary and secondary palates. Clefts can be induced in rodents under a number of experimental conditions (e.g. cortisone injection, excess vitamin A administration), though it has yet to be shown whether similar aetiological factors can produce clefts in humans.

If an aetiological factor associated with cleft formation is introduced late in development, its effect may be comparatively mild. Thus, only the soft palate may be affected, the mildest form of cleft involving just the uvula. If, however, the aetiological factor is introduced early in development, the resulting cleft may be more severe. It may extend anteriorly in the midline to affect the hard palate and, in the severest of cases, may pass out laterally between the primary and secondary palates to involve bilaterally the alveolar arches.

Considerable research has been undertaken to elucidate the mechanism of palatal shelf elevation, though the precise cause remains unclear. Many theories have been put forward and these can broadly be divided into two groups. One group holds that the shelves play a passive role, being elevated by the activity of extrinsic factors such as movement of the tongue, growth of the mandible or changes in the angulation of the cranial base. The alternative view is that shelf elevation is due to some intrinsic property of the shelves themselves, perhaps being related to differential growth, vascular changes, contraction associated with connective tissue elements or binding of water to ground substance.

Chapter 2

Anatomy

B.K.B. Berkovitz

A feature which distinguishes man from other animals is his development of language, using speech as a system of communication. A prerequisite for this would be a large brain to process, integrate and store the enormous amounts of information needed. Indeed, the acquisition of language is probably the most complex sensorimotor development in the individual's life. Considerable areas within the cerebral hemispheres are involved in the sensory, perceptual and motor aspects of speech. Human language appears to be learnt in a well-defined chronological sequence, the child requiring adequate visual, tactile and audible stimuli and the necessary intelligence.

Sounds are initially produced in the larynx by the coordinated movements of abdominal, thoracic and laryngeal muscles (*Fig.* 2.1). Subsequent modification of laryngeal sound to produce meaningful speech occurs principally within the pharyngeal, oral and nasal cavities. It will be noted that activity associated with speech utilizes mechanisms which serve other and more vital functions in the human body, namely respiration, swallowing and chewing.

The sound generated at the larynx carries a very limited range of speech information; the fundamental laryngeal note is of a thin and reedy quality. *Articulation* refers to the mechanism whereby laryngeal sound is modified within resonating chambers by the activity of organs such as the lips, tongue and soft palate to produce speech.

The *resonators* of the human voice are those air-filled spaces situated above and below the vocal cords to which sound waves have access. By a process of resonance or sympathetic vibration, the resonators act as acoustic filters, amplifying selected frequencies and attenuating others, thus enhancing and modifying the basic sound produced by the larynx. The most important are the supraglottic resonators, though subglottic resonators

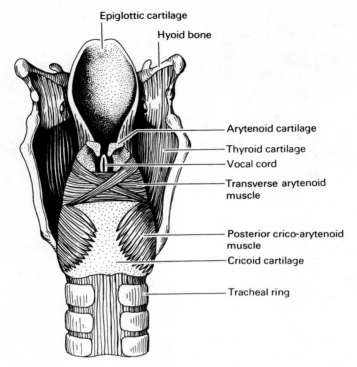

Epiglottic cartilage

Hyoid bone

Arytenoid cartilage

Thyroid cartilage

Vocal cord

Transverse arytenoid muscle

Posterior crico-arytenoid muscle

Cricoid cartilage

Tracheal ring

Fig. 2.1. The larynx viewed from behind.

comprising the tracheal and thoracic cavities presumably make some contribution. The supraglottic resonators comprise the laryngeal space above the vocal cords (the vestibule, middle part and sinus), the pharynx (oro-, naso-, and laryngo-pharynx), oral and nasal cavities and the para-nasal sinuses (*Figs* 2.2 and 2.3). Within the naso-pharynx may be seen the opening of the eustachian tube which connects the pharynx with the middle ear (*Fig.* 2.3). Spread of infection from the pharynx may cause otitis media, which may eventually affect hearing. The presence of adenoids within the naso-pharynx in excessive amounts may also affect speech, giving it a characteristic denasal tone.

It is the considerable alterations in both size and shape that can occur within the supraglottic resonators which allows for the diversity of sound. In the case of the tongue, bodily movement is carried out principally by the extrinsic group of muscles, while change in shape is due mainly to the action of intrinsic muscles. During speech, both groups are active. Extrinsic and intrinsic muscles are supplied by the hypoglossal nerve. The extrinsic muscles are illustrated in *Fig.* 2.4, and arise from structures outside the substance of the tongue. The genioglossus muscle (arising from the upper genial tubercle of the inner surface of the mandible in the midline) pulls

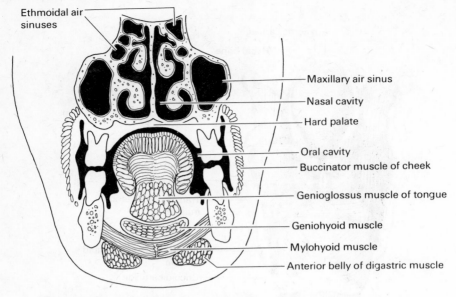

Fig. 2.2. Coronal section through head, showing position of resonators.

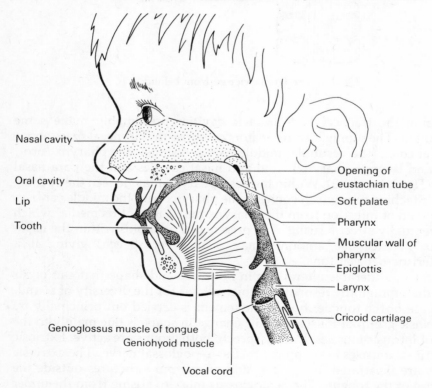

Fig. 2.3. Sagittal section through the head, showing position of supraglottic resonators.

the tongue forwards. The hyoglossus muscle (arising from the greater horn of the hyoid bone) depresses the tongue. The styloglossus muscle (arising near the tip of the styloid process) pulls the tongue upwards and backwards. Another muscle sometimes grouped with the extrinsic muscles is the

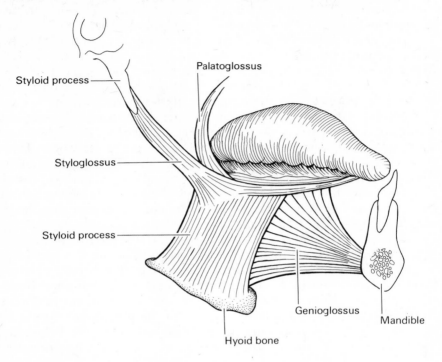

Fig. 2.4. Diagram showing extrinsic muscles of tongue.

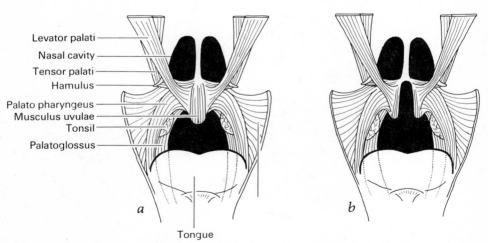

Fig. 2.5. Soft palate seen from behind. *a*, Normal. *b*, Cleft palate.

palatoglossus which lies in the anterior pillar of the fauces (*Figs* 2.4 and 2.5). Though it can elevate the root of the tongue, functionally and developmentally it should be considered a muscle of the palate (hence its innervation by the pharyngeal plexus). The mylohyoid muscle which lies in the floor of the mouth assists in elevating the tongue. The intrinsic muscles lie completely within the substance of the tongue. There are longitudinal, transverse and vertical fibre groups arranged in an interlacing network. When the longitudinal fibres contract, the tongue shortens and the tip may be raised. When the transverse fibres contract, the tongue narrows and elongates and a trough may form on the dorsal surface. Contraction of the vertical fibres causes the tongue to flatten and broaden.

The soft palate is suspended from the back of the hard palate, separating the oral and nasal parts of the pharynx (*Fig.* 2.3). For the majority of sounds, the nasal cavities and naso-pharynx are closed off by elevation of the soft palate against the posterior wall of the pharynx. The degree of elevation varies between sounds. However, for the sounds 'm', 'n' and 'ng', resonance is produced in the naso-pharynx and nasal cavities by depression of the soft palate and closure of the mouth. The muscles comprising the palate are illustrated in *Fig.* 2.5*a*. Apart from the tensor palati (which is supplied by the mandibular nerve), the muscles of the soft palate are supplied by the accessory nerve via the pharyngeal plexus. The most important is the levator palati, which, as the name suggests, elevates the soft palate. This muscle arises primarily from the petrous part of the temporal bone and enters the soft palate above the upper border of the superior constrictor. Additional activity of the latter muscle, of the palatopharyngeus and of the musculus uvulae assists in sealing off the naso-pharynx. When the soft palate is depressed, the levator palati muscles relax and additional active

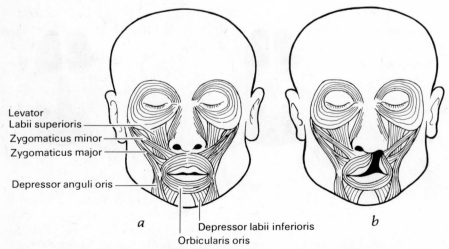

Levator Labii superioris
Zygomaticus minor
Zygomaticus major
Depressor anguli oris
a
Depressor labii inferioris
Orbicularis oris
b

Fig. 2.6. Muscles of facial expression. *a*, Normal. *b*, Cleft lip.

movement is possibly due to the palatoglossus muscles. When the nasal cavities cannot be sealed off during speech, as for example in the presence of a cleft of the palate or of a neurological disorder, there is a resulting nasal escape of air and an inability to build up intra-oral air pressure. This manifests itself in the form of vowels having a hypernasal quality and consonants being weak and muffled.

Like the tongue, the lips are comprised of both extrinsic and intrinsic muscles, all of which are supplied by the facial nerve. Among the extrinsic group are the buccinator, zygomaticus, levator and depressor anguli oris, levator labii superioris and depressor labii inferioris muscles (*Fig. 2.6a.*). The presence of clefts or conditions where the facial nerve is damaged may affect the production of certain sounds (e.g. bi-labials). Because the teeth play an important role in articulation, dental abnormalities of the anterior teeth may be associated with speech defects, particularly with reference to sounds such as 's' and 'z'.

ANATOMY OF THE CLEFT LIP

The muscles comprising the orbicularis oris of the lips are unable to attach to each other, as mesenchyme from which they develop fails to penetrate between the layers of the maxillary processes. Instead, they become attached to the nearest adjacent fixed point.

In the case of a unilateral cleft, the lateral side muscles sweep up towards the alar base with some fibres gaining attachment to the lip mucosa along the side of the cleft. On the medial side, the bulk of fibres sweep up towards the nasal spine and the base of the columella (*Fig. 2.6b*). In the bilateral cleft lip, mesenchyme does not penetrate the processes from either side. As no muscle develops from the medial nasal process, there is no muscle behind the prolabial skin, nor does prolabial skin have any hair follicles, so skin from it can be used to build up a deficiency of tissue in the columella. Indeed, it has been argued that all the prolabial skin belongs in the columella. However, a good operation for the bilateral cleft lip has not yet been devised which does not use at least part of the prolabial skin for the lip.

The abnormal insertion of the orbicularis oris pulls the medial and lateral crura of the alar cartilage outwards from the cleft and makes it fall like a visor down across the opening of the nasal passage.

ANATOMY OF THE CLEFT PALATE

When the muscles of the palate are unable to attach to each other across the midline of the cleft, they become re-orientated towards a fixed point and stream towards the half of the posterior nasal spine of their side of the cleft (*Fig. 2.5b*). The palatine aponeurosis also retracts laterally under the pull of the tensor palati, whose inserting tendon it is. Like the lip muscle, some fibres still have a normal insertion into the oral mucosa, where they produce a definite dimple as the palate lifts and are thought to be derived from levator palati.

Descriptions of the precise arrangement of the muscles differ from one investigation to another, and may represent individual variation between the specimens dissected. These variations are frequently seen in normal patients as indicated by the problem of contracture of the velopharyngeal isthmus when seen endoscopically during speech.

Chapter 3

Classification

I.S. Hathorn

The clinical problem of cleft lip and palate has been the subject of a number of complex classifications over the years. The problem is, however, so varied that only a broad classification is appropriate. The most useful classification is descriptive in nature, and splits the palate into its various anatomical areas (*Fig.* 3.1*a*).

INCIDENCE : All clefts, approximately 1 in 600.

1. CLEFT LIP

Right or left with or without involvement of the alveolus − CL.

The cleft may be right or left sided. It may be minimal, causing only a notch on the lip, or more extensive affecting the lip and alveolus.

INCIDENCE : 25 per cent.

2. UNILATERAL CLEFT LIP AND PALATE

Right or left − UCLP (*Fig.* 3.1*b*).

This cleft passes either left or right of the premaxilla, through the incisive foramen, and back through the hard and soft palate. This splits the palate into major (hard palate and premaxilla) and minor (hard palate only) segments. There is a variable displacement of these segments, depending on the muscle forces which apply during development.

INCIDENCE : 40 per cent.

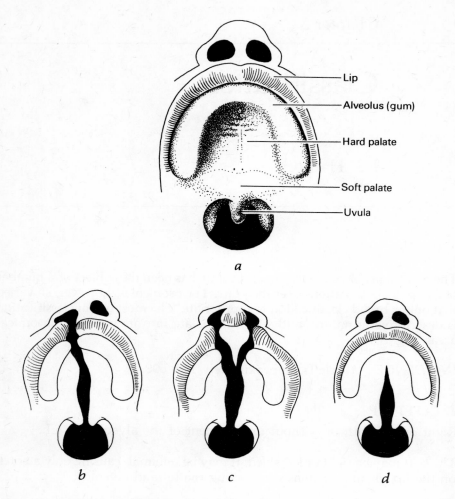

Fig. 3.1. *a*, Normal palate; *b*, Right unilateral cleft lip and palate; *c*, Bilateral cleft lip and palate; *d*, Cleft palate.

3. BILATERAL CLEFT LIP AND PALATE

BCLP (*Fig. 3.1c*).

This cleft passes down both sides of the premaxilla, through the incisive foramen, and through hard and soft palate. Due to the lack of lip control on the premaxilla, this segment is often very prominent at birth.

INCIDENCE : 10 per cent.

4. CLEFT PALATE
CP *(Fig. 3.1d)*.

The cleft of palate may extend forwards to the incisive foramen, leaving quite a wide midline cleft. The extent of this cleft can vary in a posterior direction down to a cleft of soft palate only. It is important to note that included in this group is the submucous cleft, which involves clefting of the muscle layer only in the soft palate, and exhibits little or no outward sign of cleft. The method of checking this cleft clinically is to feel the posterior border of the hard palate. Usually there will be an obvious notch in the midline where the muscles have failed to attach.

INCIDENCE : 25 per cent.

5. PIERRE-ROBIN SYNDROME

This is a syndrome which includes the cleft of the hard and soft palate (CP). It has a classic presenting triad.
   1. Cleft of hard and soft palate
   2. Retrognathia
   3. Respiratory distress
   To be diagnosed as Pierre – Robin it is necessary to fulfil all three criteria. The receding lower jaw causes the tongue to be held backwards towards the pharyngeal wall, and this is the main cause of the respiratory distress.

Chapter 4

Primary repair of the cleft lip and palate

R.W. Pigott

There is a world-wide trend to repair congenital deformities at younger and younger ages as the nature of the deformity is better understood, as the general health of babies improves and as anaesthetic techniques become safer. While some deformities must be operated upon at birth if the baby is to survive, others, like cleft lip and palate, allow the team to choose a pattern of care which they consider promises the best possible result from the many alternatives open.

The fact that there are such a lot of differences between individual patients in the severity of their cleft and their own potential to grow, means that the team must wait some twenty or twenty-five years to see the final result of enough patients to assess the overall outcome of their plan. If one realizes that this is most of the practising lifetime of a consultant, it will be appreciated that progress must be slow.

THE PROBLEM OF THE CLEFT LIP AND NOSE

The Lip

The cleft lip is not just separated, as with a knife. Repair is complicated by a variable amount of missing tissue, worst in the lower third of the lip. There are several excellent methods for correcting it. However, the amount of tissue available to the surgeon and the way in which each scar heals are at least as important as the technique chosen.

The Nose

The muscles which should be joined across the lip are forced to find another anchorage. They become attached to the ends of the area of tissue that forms the nostril, pulling it down like a visor. Even the tiniest web of skin bridging the cleft will reduce the deformity of the nose a great deal. The muscles

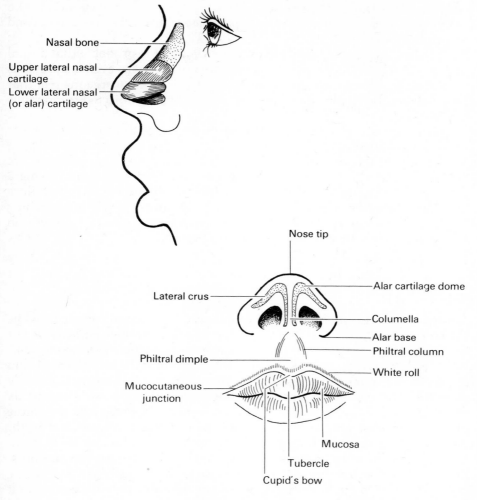

Nasal bone

Upper lateral nasal cartilage

Lower lateral nasal (or alar) cartilage

Nose tip

Alar cartilage dome

Lateral crus

Columella

Alar base

Philtral column

Philtral dimple

White roll

Mucocutaneous junction

Mucosa

Tubercle

Cupid's bow

Fig. 4.1. The external anatomy of the lip and nose.

will be joined to each other in the cleft lip repair and immediately a considerable correction of the nose occurs. There are more delicate abnormalities of the alar cartilages (*Fig.* 4.1), which give the tip of the nose its shape, and some surgeons believe that these should be put into a better position at the first operation. Others believe that the parts can be put into the correct position more easily and reliably when the nose has had time to grow, perhaps just before the child goes to primary school.

There is an increasing trend towards freeing the alar cartilage from the bone at the first operation, because many surgeons are reporting their experience that the children look more normal earlier in life, need less operations overall and are teased less as they grow. But it should also be said that another decade may have to pass before this will be proved beyond reasonable doubt.

The nose changes dramatically at puberty and it is probable that a final operation will be necessary for some children in the teens, even if a previous correction has been performed. Because of this, some surgeons feel that they will get the best result if the nose has not been subjected to previous operations.

The septum is always bent in children with a cleft through the bone at the gum and hard part of the palate. This will produce a variable degree of blockage of the nose on one or both sides and once again surgeons are not yet certain about how early it can be straightened without risking a reduction of the growth of the bone in the middle of the face. A failure of the middle part of the face to grow normally can occur without touching the septum, so it is almost impossible to separate the effect of surgery on the septum from an inherent failure to develop.

THE PALATE

The hard palate is supported by bony shelves with mucosal coverings, while the soft palate consists of muscle with mucosal covering. Early repair of the cleft of the hard and soft palate is undertaken by many surgeons, with two main objectives: to make the control of food in the mouth easier and to keep it out of the nose, and to give the child as near a normal anatomy as possible by the time it starts experimenting with sounds at three to six months of age. To achieve this, many surgeons are operating on the whole palate in the first year and some under six months, a few even at birth. However, there appears to be proportionately less tissue available at birth, in the soft palate especially, and this develops well in the next few months. Dissection of the structures of the palate also becomes easier as they become larger. Some delay in operation may also be desirable to make certain that the baby has no other congenital problem such as heart disease which could affect the safety of an operation.

Each type of cleft (e.g. unilateral, bilateral) needs some modification to the general plan of which there have been two main schools, both dedicated to the belief that their operation was designed to allow the palate to close the nose from the mouth at the right moments and so permit the patient to develop normal speech. The palate had to be long enough and, above all, mobile. One school (Von Langenbeck) simply moves tissue sideways to join it up with a simple scar down the midline. By delicate surgery, a mobile palate could be achieved, but no attempt was made at lengthening the palate. The other school, considering that often there would be a shortage of tissue in the soft palate, so that the palate would not reach the posterior pharyngeal wall, sought to lengthen the palate by moving the mucoperiosteum of the hard palate backwards as well as towards the midline. This operation was developed by a Parisian surgeon, Victor Veau, in the late nineteenth century and is still widely followed. His reasoning persuaded many surgeons at the turn of the century to abandon the Langenbeck operation, but continuing studies have left doubt of the supremacy of one procedure over the other from the speech point of view. It has also been shown by several workers that Veau's technique increases the amount of raw area over the hard palate bone and may hold back forward growth of the face to a measurable degree.

Another approach to the problem has been developed in the last twenty-five years, to try to reduce the amount of collapse of the alveolar arch which occurs to a greater or lesser extent in almost all children whose cleft is completely through the alveolar bone. This is partly due to the deficiency of tissue, both bony and soft. In addition, the bone itself may have reduced potential to grow, particularly at the margins of the cleft. So when skin, muscle and mucosa are stretched towards each other as in the repair of the lip and soft palate, they exert relentless forces on the bone which restrict its ability to grow naturally. Repairing the cleft involves separating the periosteum from the bone. Together with the mucosa and the tissue between, they form a living sheet which can be moved across the cleft and sutured to the opposite side. In doing so, an area of bone is left open at the sides, and this area is healed by cells from the edge of the mucosa and periosteum. But tissue thus formed does not have a normal blood supply and so is not able to develop as well. These observations have resulted in a policy, more widely practised on the continent of Europe than in Britain, to repair the cleft in the soft palate early, but to defer repairing the hard palate until the bony tissue has had longer to develop. In this regime, the hard palate will be left for five to seven years and it has been observed that the cleft between the edges of the bony palate shelves will frequently become narrower in this time, so that the edges almost touch. Joining the mucosa in such cases can be done with almost no displacement of the precious mucoperiosteum. In other children, the gap may remain quite wide, but it is believed that the bone has more ability to resist the collapsing forces generated by contracting scar tissue. Prior to surgery, some of the children will learn to cope without getting food and drink into the nose. Others will need to wear an obturator to prevent this, and to prevent air escaping into the nose when they talk. A more difficult matter to decide is whether the remaining hole in the hard palate affects the development of speech. Some children will have difficulty in developing good speech patterns anyway, due to quite unrelated factors such as hearing and intelligence, and perhaps most of all the amount of interest and help families give their children. So the answer lies in finding the proportions of good and bad speakers and it continues to be very difficult to know whether the price paid in speech quality is compensated for by better facial growth and appearance. A clear answer to this is not yet available.

TIMING OF THE OPERATION

This varies quite widely, so it will be found that surgeons will choose a time from within twenty-four hours of birth to up to six or even twelve months after for this first operation. The advantages of early operation include the reduction of the enormously distressing time that parents must suffer the appearance of their child and the fact that in very young children the bone can be moulded quite easily, so that joining the lip together is easily achieved. Other surgeons prefer to wait for a few months to allow the baby to grow bigger and stronger. With more tissue available, these surgeons feel that a more precise operation can be done. In the meantime, it may be decided that pre-surgical orthopaedics can be carried out to assist the surgical closure of the lip (Chapter 6).

ADMISSION TO HOSPITAL

The hospital will give the family as much warning as possible to bring their child in. The actual warning depends on factors such as the likelihood of a run of emergencies filling beds, so that cancellations would occur unacceptably often if a long warning is given, or there might be an outbreak of measles or other infection which would make it dangerous for a child who was not immune. Even an outbreak of 'flu' among the ward nurses might make it unwise for children to be admitted. On the other hand, parents who know that their child was to be admitted by a certain age should certainly enquire if more than a month or two has passed after the proposed date. Information will be sent on how to find the hospital (which may often be a different one from where their child was originally seen by the surgeon), what to bring in, visiting hours, the availability of mothers' accommodation in or nearby the unit.

TESTS ON ADMISSION

Routine tests of blood and throat and nose swabs may be needed before the operation. The results can take up to three days to come through. The time is not wasted, in that the family will get to know the ward routines before the operation day. The blood is tested for anaemia and the nose and throat swabs for the presence of bacteria which could cause infection and spoil healing.

THE OPERATION DAY

The baby will be starved for several hours before the operation, to make sure the stomach is empty. This is to be sure that if the baby was to vomit, there would be nothing which could irritate the lungs while protective reflexes are weakened by the anaesthetic. Pre-medication as a drink or by injection will be given an hour or so before operation. It will sometimes be necessary to make up the lost feed by intravenous infusion during the time the baby is in the theatre.

THE OPERATION

The Lip

The natural landmarks of the lip and nose are shown in *Fig.* 4.1. All three layers, skin, mucosa and muscle, are carefully freed from the base of the nose and the alveolar bone and each layer joined to the opposite side. The way the tissues come down into alignment is shown in *Fig.* 4.2*a* for the widely used Millard operation and two other common ways of 'filling' the missing triangle of skin are shown in *Fig.* 4.2*b, c*. In principle, there is a deficiency of tissue and so the less that is thrown away the better. The Millard scar follows a natural ridge (philtral ridge) and its zig-zag is hidden up under the nose. The Tennison operation has its zig-zag in the more obvious lower third of the lip, so, if it does not heal well, the extra low scarring is more obvious, but it produces a very nice fullness in the lower third of the lip. Other patterns of operations are used, but these two produce consistently good results for many surgeons.

Two other corrections may be made before joining the lip. The floor of the nose may be rebuilt through the alveolar gap using tissue from each side of the gap to make the floor of the nose. The floor of the nose is sometimes reinforced underneath with mucosa which can be spared from the lip. The feet of the arch of the cartilage which makes the shape of the nose tip, are pulled apart like doing the splits and falling forwards at the same time, by the abnormal muscle pull. This is partially corrected as the lip muscle comes together. If the surgeon decides to further correct it, this will require extra cuts inside the nose to free the cartilage from the bony edges of the cleft.

Bilateral Cleft Lip

The two sides of a cleft lip may be joined at one operation in most cases, but some surgeons consider that it is safer to allow one side to heal before embarking on the other side. Symmetry is harder to achieve in non-simultaneous repairs, but more may be done to correct the nose deformity. It is a very complicated operation and each surgeon tends to feel at home with one combination of operations. Two or even three stages may be planned over the first few years of life, quite apart from any revision operations that may be required to correct asymmetry. It is also much more difficult to make a bilateral cleft lip repair look normal; apart from the severity of the deformity, the surgeon has nothing to compare with as he does in a unilateral cleft. One pattern of repair is shown in *Fig.* 4.3.

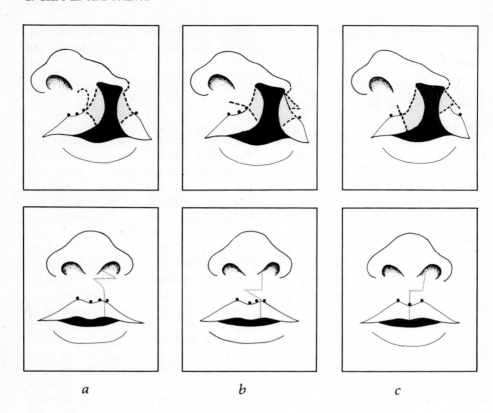

a   b   c

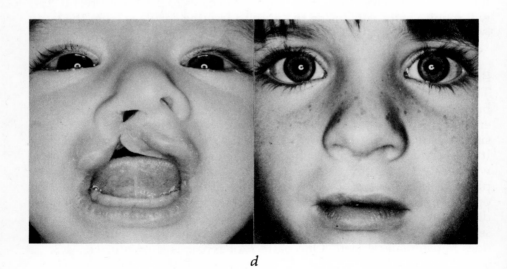

d

Fig. 4.2.

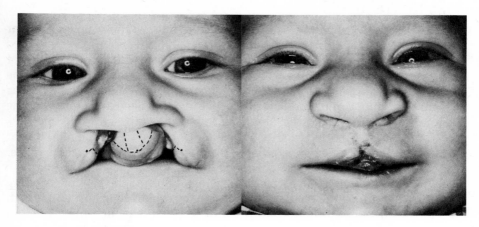

Fig. 4.3. The Millard bilateral lip repair. A narrow strip of prolabial skin is marked to represent the philtrum. The rest is stored beneath the nostrils. The muscle is united behind the philtrum. The tip of the nose is still flattened and must wait for the next stage of the operation (*see* Chapter 5). The mucosa making the philtrum under the cupid's bow all comes from the lateral elements.

AFTER OPERATION

The hospital will have a routine to protect the lip while it is healing. To prevent the baby irritating the fresh cut by sucking its thumb, cardboard cylinders may be bandaged round the arms to keep them straight. Spoon feeding may be considered safer than bottle or breast for a few days until the scar is stronger. Stitches will be removed at intervals over a week. Sometimes a pack may be put inside the nose and removed during the first week; also stitches may be tied over a little roll of gauze to help shape the nostril.

Fig. 4.2. *a.* The Millard rotation-advancement operation. The cupid's bow is tilted up the side of the cleft. It will be rotated down, with a curved cut up under the columella. The gap left is filled with a wedge of skin, muscle and mucosa from the upper part of the lateral side of the cleft.

    b. The Tennison triangular flap operation. The cut to correct the cupid's bow is made low on the lip. The gap is filled with a triangle of skin, muscle and mucosa from the lower end of the lateral lip element.

    c. The Le Mesurier operation. The natural cupid's bow is ignored and a new one made by bending down flaps from both sides of the cleft. The operation is not performed so often nowadays as the long-term results have been rather unpredictable.

    d. Millard repair, before operation and 5 years later.

THE PALATE REPAIR

The cleft palate is repaired in one or two layers, so there will be a scar more or less straight down the middle of the palate. The tissue may be moved towards this without tension by making cuts out at the sides of the roof of the mouth to relax the tissue during healing. These raw areas have bone beneath them (*Fig.* 4.4), so the defects do not go into the nose. The areas heal up in about three weeks with surprisingly little scarring, but some irregularity of the roof of the mouth is to be expected. This becomes less with time. Often, dissolving stitches are used, but some surgeons feel that silk stitches are more comfortable to the patient while they are in place, even though they have to be removed under a general anaesthetic.

It will be necessary to keep a child in hospital until the risk of bleeding is over, to supervise the feeding, using first liquid and then soft diet which does not need to be broken up in the mouth before swallowing. A raised temperature after palate operation is quite common and often no real cause is found. The edges of the cuts almost always look rather yellow and messy. This does not necessarily mean that anything is wrong. Swelling above the palate from the surgery can block the eustachian tube and may need treatment.

FOLLOW-UP

After the primary surgery is over, the baby will be able to develop without further surgery, assuming that there have been no complications. For some children, nothing further is ever required, but for most children with complete clefts, one or more secondary operation will be needed and these are covered in Chapter 5.

COMPLICATIONS

The Lip Operation

Breakdown of the repair. With a healthy baby and modern surgery, this is rare, but sometimes, especially in bilateral clefts, there is such a shortage of tissue that the repair is extremely tight and the tension causes death of the tissue around the stitches, which come loose, and this is often associated with infection. It is usually impossible to resuture the lip at this time, so the child must be allowed to grow bigger before a second repair is attempted.

Hypertrophic Scar. Many babies make very good scars on the lip. A few may be less lucky and for reasons that are not understood, the scar becomes thick, red and short, pulling the lip margin up. This change will settle very slowly over a variable period from six months to six years. At present, there is nothing that can be done to get over the problem, but where the

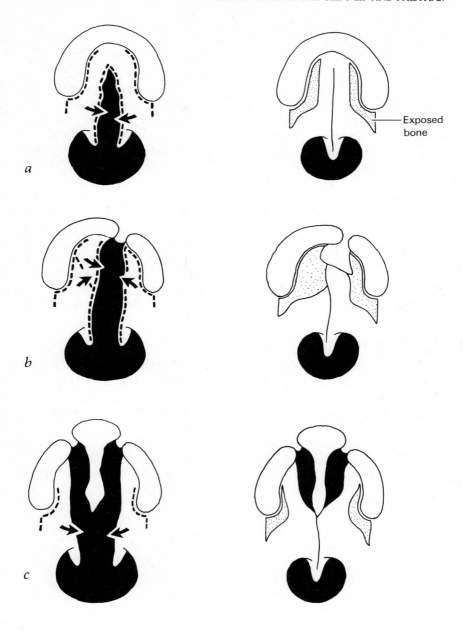

Exposed bone

a

b

c

Fig. 4.4. *a.* A cleft of the secondary palate closed by the Langenbeck technique.

    b. A complete unilateral cleft through the alveolus, closed by the Veau technique.

    c. A bilateral complete cleft closed by the delayed hard palate repair technique.

lip has been long enough at operation, it will eventually be long enough again when the scar settles.

The Nose
Blockage of the nose (stenosis). This may be due to the same sort of scar formation as described for the lip, or sometimes just due to an inadequate amount of lining mucosa. It produces very few problems for the child. Most often, mother notices that when the child has a cold, the nostril does not run. If obstruction occurs on both sides, children can be very distressed by not being able to breathe through the nose at night.

Sleep apnoea. A very rare, but important, type of breathing difficulty occurs when a child has a blocked nose and also has a tongue that will not stay down from the palate during sleep. The child fights for breath with gasping breathing and when it has got enough air to be going on with, it falls deeper asleep, the tongue rises to block the mouth and breathing stops for many seconds until the child half wakes again. Such children do not get a good night's sleep and even growth and intelligence can be affected. It is vital that the surgeon in charge of the child is informed urgently so that the problem can be investigated and treated.

The Palate
Fistulae. A fistula is a hole from mouth to nose where part of the cleft failed to heal. The treatment of fistulae is covered in Chapter 5. Soft palate fistulae mean that the muscles across the palate have separated as well as a breakdown in mucosa and it is vital to repair them as soon as the tissues are healthy again, so that normal air control develops.

Failure of the palate to work properly cannot often be diagnosed with confidence before the age of two to three years, when the child will have enough words upon which to make a judgement. Further surgery for the palate incompetence, as it is called, may be required.

Chapter 5

Secondary surgery

R.W. Pigott

The same variation of treatment plan which is practised between different cleft palate teams in the initial surgery is inevitably carried on into secondary surgery.

In part, the need for secondary surgery demonstrates the shortcomings of initial surgery to correct all the innumerable facets of the cleft lip and palate child's deformity. In part, secondary surgery will be needed because certain problems do not make their appearance until later. For example, the adult nose shape develops in the teens. When the inherited shape is superimposed on an unpredictable amount of underdevelopment of the underlying maxillary bone, due to the cleft and also due to the corrective surgery, it may be seen that final correction must await the stabilization of these factors. It must also await corrective movements on the underlying bone and teeth which may be undertaken by the orthodontist in the early teens and major surgery on the maxilla which may be undertaken in the late teens.

It has been considered that operation on a tissue early on may impair its growth potential by damaging its blood supply or restricting its growth by scar tissue. For example, it was considered on the grounds of facial development studies, that the septum of the nose had a major role in pushing forward the whole of the middle third of the face. This special growth phase was considered to be over by the age of seven, so children would have to wait until at least seven years of age before the septum could be straightened safely. Concepts of facial growth have changed considerably and it is no longer widely accepted that the septum influences the total maxillary growth, but too early or extensive an operation on the septum can still retard forward growth of the nose tip itself. So a relative contra-indication still exists for too radical early septal surgery.

THE LIP

Children start to be self-aware at about three or four years of age. So play groups or nurseries will be the first place in which unfavourable reactions may be experienced. However, the groups are small and as yet unskilled at exploiting unfavourable characteristics in others. By primary school age, around five years, these reactions are much more strongly developed and by secondary school the chances of being thrown into a large new group of potentially hostile children are higher still. These milestones may be taken as indications for adjustments to be made before the child joins a new group to minimize the risk of harassment.

Where certain improvement is likely, surgeons will usually encourage early adjustment. If the results are more doubtful and the chances of yet another operation are high, it may be felt necessary to advise waiting, despite the appreciation of the very real distress that the decision will inflict on children in their most vulnerable years.

For each basic operation, there is a group of secondary corrections which may be used, too numerous to detail here, but an example is shown in *Fig.* 5.1. Lip scars may need to be lengthened or shortened. Wide scars may mean a weak muscle repair beneath. The cupid's bow line between skin and mucosa of the lip may need to be resculptured and the thickness of the mucosa built up or thinned.

In practice, lip revision by itself is a small procedure, likely to require less than a week in hospital, causing very little pain, and most children will be strongly enough healed to return to school in two weeks and play games after three or four weeks.

Two specific problems may be discussed more fully.

Columella Lengthening

In the case of a bilateral cleft lip, it is not possible to make all the corrections at one stage, so it may be decided to unite the lip at the first stage and leave the nose until the second.

In one method of achieving this, all the skin of the central segment of the lip (prolabium) is united to the lateral lip elements at the first stage (*Fig.* 5.2). At a later stage, the outer part of this skin is taken out of the lip as two fork-like prongs (Millard's forked flap operation) based on the columella and used to lengthen the columella, which is desperately short in many bilateral cleft lips.

Alternatively, the lateral parts of the prolabial skin may be taken up and 'stored' horizontally beneath the alar bases at the first operation, so that the vertical lip scars do not need to be touched again (*Fig.* 5.3). The stored skin is then moved up into the columella at the second operation. This can be done a few weeks to several years after the initial operation and the tendency now is to wait several years as the long-term result is more stable. The advantage of this is that it has been observed that scars made in infants

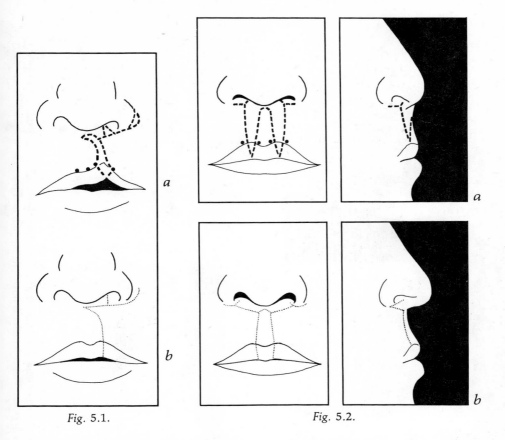

Fig. 5.1.   Fig. 5.2.

Fig. 5.1. *a*. Short lip scar due to inadequate rotation and advancement at the primary operation. *b*. Re-rotation and further advancement to give full length scar, careful alignment of the mucocutaneous junction and mucosal advancement to fill out the lip mucosa.

Fig. 5.2. *a*. All the prolabial skin has been kept in the lip. The lip muscle has not been united across behind the skin, which becomes stretched. *b*. The lip muscle has been united. All prolabial skin, apart from that which is needed to make the normal lip philtrum, has been turned up into the columella of the nose to allow it to project normally. Lateral lip mucosa has been united in the midline.

not infrequently fade to a degree almost never achieved in older children. It is certainly very distressing to find that the revised vertical lip scars behave badly after a later operation, becoming thick and red (hypertrophic).

Abbe Flap
The upper lip is frequently short of tissue and consequently the normal lower lip may look protuberant. A drooping lower lip can look sullen, even pugnacious. The upper lip may be lying on a bony maxilla which lacks

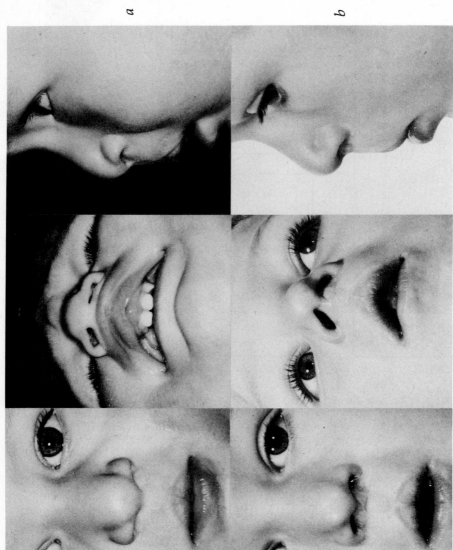

Fig. 5.3. This illustration shows the second stage correction of the child seen in Chapter 4. *a.* The lip scars are well-healed and the stored skin can be seen. From below, the columella is very short and from the side the nose tip is flat. *b.* The extra tissue was moved into the columella at 4.5 years. The columella is now long enough and the nose tip projects normally in the side view.

the proper amount of forward projection. In some patients, in addition, the original lip repair may not have produced a normal cupid's bow.

In such cases, a very satisfactory solution may be achieved by transferring a wedge of the full thickness of the lower lip on a bridge of tissue into a midline cut on the upper lip, ignoring the old lip scars completely (*Fig.* 5.4). The bridge of tissue divides the mouth opening into two for ten to fourteen days while the tissue picks up a new blood supply, after which the bridge is divided and both top and bottom lip scars completed. The patient has to have a liquid diet during this time, but may be able to go home for at least part of the time. The lower lip is thus tightened and the upper lip loosened, with a very considerable improvement overall.

Sometimes, the whole scarred centre of the upper lip may be used to lengthen the columella of the nose and the Abbe flap used to replace the philtrum.

NOSE REVISION

Where a nose is symmetrical, the lip scar may well be taken to be the result of an accident and all the inhibitions arising from the awareness of congenital deformity are avoided. The nasal deformity is thus enormously important. It almost invariably becomes worse with age, is very complex in its three-dimensional components and is widely considered to be difficult or impossible to correct perfectly. Many proponents of early attempts at correction have been disappointed by the rate of relapse to the original deformity and teach the wisdom of waiting until the parts are larger and easier to manage technically. Nevertheless, a wave of opinion is gathering in favour of early correction. It has been shown that, overall, less operations are required to achieve a certain standard of result. In the meantime, early alleviation of the disfigurement makes life easier for the child in these most critical years.

Nose Tip

Secondary operations will include balancing operations to the tip. It can be observed quite often that the cleft side will not project so far forward and the nostril rim will hang down. From below, the cleft side nostril apex will be too far back and the cleft side alar base will be too far back, too high or too low. Surgeons learn a group of procedures to correct these. Very often, all the tissue required is present and simply needs to be adjusted. Sometimes a shortage of bone, cartilage, skin or mucosal lining may be present. Bone may be taken from the hip bone or a rib, cartilage from the nasal septum or from the concha of the ear through a little cut at the back, skin from the back of the ear, mucosa from the lining on one side of the nasal septum or the inside of the cheek. An example is shown in *Fig.* 5.5. Like the cleft lip, the operations are not major: discharge in less than a week, return to school in two weeks and games in four will usually be possible.

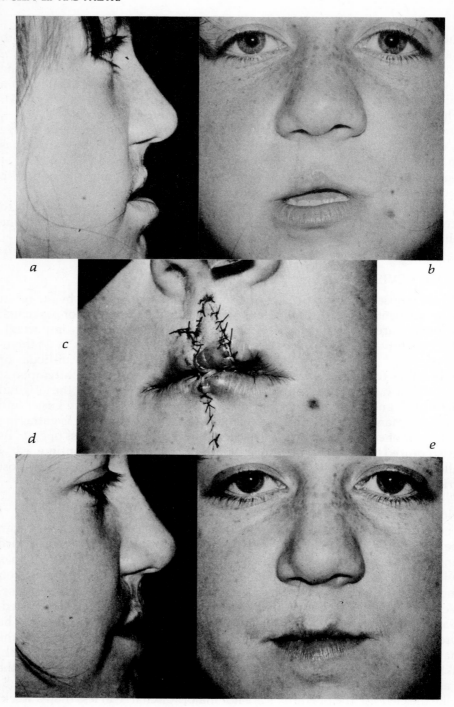

Fig. 5.4.

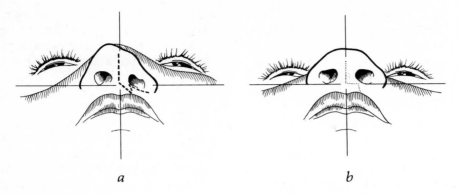

a   *b*

Fig. 5.5. a. From the front, the tip of the nose is lower on the cleft side and, from below, the dome of the nose and the alar base are both too far back. The surgical markings can be seen, by which the columella will be lengthened, sliding up some scar tissue from the old scar at the top of the lip. *b.* The alar base has been advanced with the lateral crus of the alar cartilage through a cut inside the nose. This, with the columella lengthening, gives the correct projection of the dome.

Nasal Septum

The nasal septum may be straightened from seven years onwards, when symptoms justify it. These include mouth breathing, dry mouth, noisy eating (with mouth open), headaches, catarrh, snoring and, rarely, sinusitis. Surprisingly often, children with gross obstruction do not complain. They grew up with it, after all!

The operation depends on the fact that the septal cartilage is always convex part of the way back in the cleft airway and the lower border, where it projects free from a bony crest of the vomerine bone, is dislocated into the normal nostril. Thus, both sides are blocked. The cartilage must usually be freed from the vomerine crest which is holding it in the distorted position, even after the primary distorting force of the cleft lip muscle has been realigned. It is then scored on its concave side, which makes the concavity flatten. The nasal cavities are then packed to hold the cartilage straight while it heals. It must be said that the cartilage and soft tissues have a 'memory', and may try to drift back to where they came from. So a perfect alignment is hard to achieve in all cases.

Fig. 5.4. a, b. Although the lip scar is good, the cupid's bow is distorted. From the side view, the lower lip is protuberant. *c.* The wedge of tissue from the midline of the lower lip, joned by a narrow bridge containing the artery, is inset into the midline of the old lip scar. *d, e.* After the bridge is cut (ten to fourteen days later), the cupid's bow is re-established and from the side the lip balance is correct.

Very rarely, the nasal bones are crooked and need to be broken and reset. This too can be done from age seven, but it is very rare for this to be indicated before the teens, and usually it can wait for the final correction after orthodontic and surgical correction of the maxilla and mandible.

THE HARD PALATE AND ALVEOLUS

The secondary surgery may become necessary if there are symptoms due to a fistula. This can be in front of, through or behind the alveolus, or in the main hard palate. Quite large fistulae may cause no symptoms, while pinhole fistulae may be a considerable nuisance. Symptoms include fluids coming down the nose. Ice cream and chocolate, which are melted against the palate by the tongue to enjoy the flavour, are commonly mentioned. These are highly antisocial problems. Fistulae in the hard palate may let air through during speech (*see* Chapter 7). The child may attempt to hold the tongue against the fistulae to stop the abnormal resonance, but this

Fig. 5.6. Closure of palate fistula with local tissue.

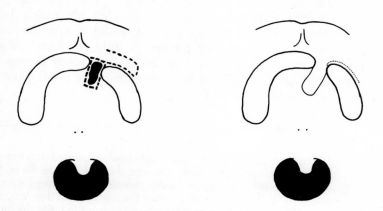

Fig. 5.7. Closure of palate fistula with buccal sulcus mucosa for oral layer cover.

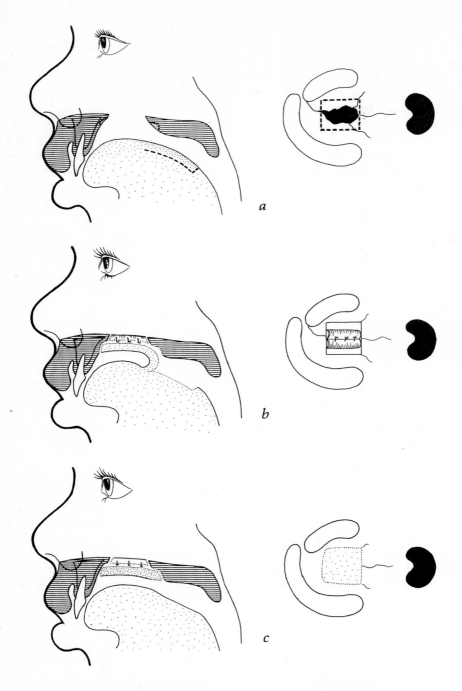

Fig. 5.8. *a*. The fistula is shown on a section of the head with the tongue flap outlined. On the roof of the mouth the inturned flaps are marked. *b*. The tongue flap is in position in the section view. The inturned flaps have been closed on the roof of the mouth. *c*. The tongue flap is shown in the roof of the mouth.

makes tremendous difficulties in articulation. The irritant effect of fluid and food in the nose may cause catarrh or a running nose.

Closure of a fistula may be done at any age, and probably the sooner the better, provided that it is causing symptoms and that suitable tissues are available. The simplest closure is with tissue of the palate adjacent to the hole (*Fig.* 5.6). This can be made to provide a lining for the nose from one side of the hole, the tissue 'flap' being hinged on the scar at the cleft margin. Needless to say, its blood supply is rather precarious. The oral layer is made by sliding a flap of mucosa sideways across the hole. The oral layer may alternatively come from inside the buccal sulcus if the fistula is in or just behind the alveolar cleft (*Fig.* 5.7). Hospital stay would be likely to be one or two weeks.

Where there is inadequate tissue, new tissues may have to be brought in. The buccal sulcus mucosa has been mentioned, but if no local tissues can be obtained, part of the top of the tongue can often be used.

A tongue flap is a trapdoor-like piece of mucosa and muscle, usually with its hinge at the front. It is designed so that it flips forward through 180° and its raw side comes to lie under the hard palate (*Fig.* 5.8). When healing is sufficiently advanced, the hinge is cut, the tongue tidied up and the hinge edge of the flap closed.

About three to seven days after the second operation, the patient may go home. Normal diet may be eaten after about two weeks. Some feeling of numbness and loss of taste may be noticed to begin with, but these sensations will come back. Tongue mobility is not interfered with and speech is not affected once the discomfort settles. Indeed, closing the fistula may improve the clarity of the speech.

THE SOFT PALATE

Fistulae of the soft palate are quite rare and surgery is most likely to be needed if the speech assessment shows that the soft palate is not performing its job of closing the nose from the mouth. Mobility and timing are both important, so a slow palate lift may be too late for the air released from the larynx through the vocal cords.

A number of operations have been devised to help the soft palate and other active muscles around the velopharyngeal isthmus to close. Two very commonly performed operations depend on different principles:

a. The posterior pharyngeal wall may be brought forward so that a short or not very mobile soft palate can then close against it. Movement of the soft palate or of tissue built onto the posterior wall, must be present for the isthmus to move from open to shut.

b. The other principle depends on providing a blockage across the centre of the isthmus by stitching a trapdoor flap of tissue from the posterior pharyngeal wall onto the soft palate. This bridge of tissue must be big enough so that movement inwards of the side walls of the pharynx can close against its sides. When the side walls relax, there must be a big enough gap for normal nasal breathing.

Either group of operations cure many patients of their problem or, at any rate, reduce the loss of air up the nose to a point where the mechanism is efficient enough for the patient to develop intelligible speech, and at the same time prevent too much resonance of air in the nose.

In order to select the operation most likely to cure a patient, some investigations may be undertaken.

X-ray Investigations

The most readily available investigation is to look at the soft palate by X-rays taken from the side of the face and neck. The maximum palate lift can be studied. Barium sulphate (contrast material — opaque to X-rays) may be instilled into the nose, so that it runs over the upper surface of the soft palate, to make a sharper picture. With barium sulphate another useful view is taken with the head thrown right back. The X-ray beam passes from beneath the jaw out at the top of the head and outlines the circumference of the isthmus. This allows the amount of side wall movement to be checked. This information can be obtained on sustained sounds such as 'e' and 's', but dynamic records from continuous speech, with a television camera and an image intensifier that use a very low dose of X-rays, permit more delicate observations to be made.

X-rays are sometimes difficult to interpret and the information can be supplemented by direct views of the isthmus from above via the nose using a naso-pharyngoscope. Measurement is not possible with this instrument used on its own, but it complements X-ray studies very well by clarifying their interpretation.

These investigations are particularly helpful where a patient has had a pharyngoplasty performed, but the result has been a disappointment. Often the cause quickly becomes apparent and a further operation can be planned with confidence of success in many cases. Certainly, hope of an improvement in any patient with unacceptable speech should never be abandoned until such investigations have provided full information on the state of the isthmus at rest and during speech efforts.

Chapter 6

Dental management

I.S. Hathorn

In the United Kingdom, the orthodontist is frequently involved with cleft lip and palate cases from birth to the final corrective phase. In orthodontic management there are three main periods, and these can be split chronologically into:

1. Pre-surgical orthopaedics.
2. Early dental management.
3. Management in the permanent dentition.

PRE-SURGICAL ORTHOPAEDICS

Pre-surgical orthopaedics is the manipulation of the maxillary bony segments by intra- and extra-oral devices fitted as soon as possible after birth. The aim in treatment should be to establish a more normal arch form. The fundamental principle of orthopaedics is that small forces continuously applied will cause the bony segments to be moved in preplanned directions. There is considerable controversy worldwide as to the benefits. Management procedures range from those who use orthopaedics up to about 3 months old, through to those who continue with maxillary manipulation up to 5-6 years old. There are also many units where pre-surgical orthopaedics is not used in any form. In this country pre-surgical orthopaedics is widely practised, and the considered benefits gained from using the technique are as below.

Aid to surgical repair of the lip and palate. Surgical repair of the lip can be made easier by closing down the gap between the lip margins. Any help in reducing the post-operative lip tension must benefit wound healing and reduce the uncontrolled forces on the developing maxilla.

Improved and redirected growth of the maxilla. It is considered by some orthodontists that pre-surgical orthopaedic repositioning of the bony segments will help in the future growth and development of the maxilla. Evidence for these claims is limited.

Improved feeding. Feeding may be helped by fitting an acrylic plate over the hard palate cleft.

Improved speech development. Speech development begins early, and it is considered that a more normal tongue position may be established early by fitting plates which cover the cleft. This may help prevent the tongue from developing a position too high and too far back in the mouth, and avoid the formation of poor speech.

Psychological support for the parents. Such support is often needed in this early phase. As pre-surgical orthopaedics demands regular visits to the orthodontist, he has the opportunity to get to know the parents well, and to give appropriate advice and support.

Pre-surgical orthopaedic treatment, where it is necessary, will be on the following lines:

In the case of the unilateral cleft lip and palate (UCLP), a plate should be fitted within the first 48 hours of life. Where the lip gap and bony cleft are wide, or the arch segments poorly positioned, an active plate or plates would then be made to mould the bony units into the desired position (*Fig. 6.1*). The first appliance to be fitted should be a passive plate with no active force on the bony segments. This allows the baby to get used to a well fitting appliance in the mouth. In particular the tongue must establish itself against the new palatal outline, and feeding can be established in a relatively trouble-free environment. It also allows the parents to become confident in feeding and caring for the baby.

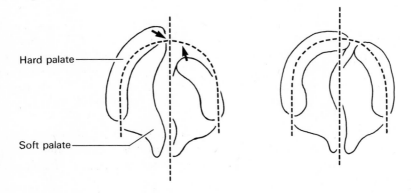

Hard palate

Soft palate

Fig. 6.1. The moulding effect seen after the use of an active plate.

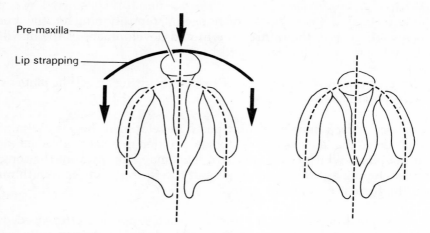

Fig. 6.2. The effect of lip strapping on the pre-maxilla.

To make an active plate a plaster model is cast from an impression of the upper jaw. This is cut and the segments moved by 1-2 mm in a predetermined way, with the aim of improving the arch shape and reducing the width of the cleft. The segments are then joined and an active appliance made from this new cast, which is then used in the mouth to mould the bony units into the desired position. The orthopaedic forces provided by the plate will come from strapping applied to wires attached to the plate onto the face or from the simple moulding function of the tongue against the plate. Further plates will be made as necessary, until the final, more normal, alignment is achieved.

In the bilateral cleft of lip and palate (BCLP) the premaxillary segment is attached to the nasal septum. This is a rapidly growing area in the newborn baby; the premaxilla is projected forwards and away from the posteriorly placed segments of the hard palate (*Fig.* 6.2). A plate may be fitted to hold the hard palate segments, or there may be a need to expand the hard palate and bring it into its normal relationship with the lower jaw. The continued forward growth of the premaxilla should be restrained by some form of lip strapping. The plate can be trimmed to allow the posterior segments to catch up by growing anteriorly. When a more normal arch form is achieved, it is usually time for surgery. The aim is to complete this alignment by about 3 months old.

Clefts of the palate (CP) may be so wide that the tongue lies within the cleft region while at rest. A plate should be fitted to prevent this. Keeping the tongue out of the cleft gives the opportunity for palatal shelf growth towards the midline.

To summarize, pre-surgical orthopaedics can certainly help surgery by realigning the bony segments and reducing the lip gap. By skilful manipulation of the plate, hard palate shelf growth can be encouraged. The long-term effect of pre-surgical orthopaedics on general maxillary growth is controversial; the effect is likely to be small. In general, pre-surgical plates are of limited value in improving feeding. Many babies feed better without a plate. In those cases, however, where the tongue lies in the cleft, there will be considerable benefit gained in both feeding and in the encouragement of lateral shelf growth.

EARLY DENTAL DEVELOPMENT

A cleft passes through the region of the lateral incisor, and will cause disturbance to the dental lamina. The main effect on the teeth is that the lateral incisor may be absent or malformed in both the deciduous and the permanent dentition.

An important objective in the management of cleft cases is the reduction of problems caused by decay. The more healthy teeth that remain when orthodontic treatment begins, the better chance the orthodontist has of achieving a good dental relationship. It is also one way of reducing visits to the dental surgeon for a patient who will see many specialists.

If the family dental practitioner advises that the fluoride content of the local water supply is inadequate, fluoride supplements in the form of drops or tablets should be given at recommended levels. In general, fluoride should be taken with the first solid food, and continued until about 10 years old. Regular visits to the dentist should begin as soon as possible, at first mainly to gain the child's confidence, but with mouth checks from the time that the deciduous dentition is established (approximately 2.5 years of age). Tooth brushing with fluoride toothpaste should also be an integral part

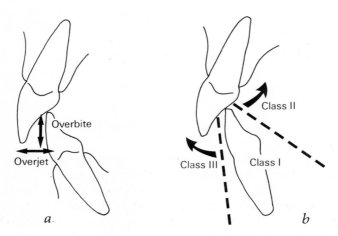

Fig. 6.3. *a.* Normal incisor relationship. *b.* Classification of incisor relationship (after Stephens and Bass).

of dental care. By these means it is possible to keep fillings to an absolute minimum.

The palatal surface of the upper incisor is divided into three parts. In the class I case the lower incisor contacts the middle part as shown (*Fig. 6.3b*). Occlusion anterior to this is class III and posterior to it class II. The latter is subdivided — division 1 cases having an overjet in excess of 3 mm and division 2 cases invariably having an excessive overbite.

Classification of Skeletal Relationship

When teeth erupt into the mouth they are influenced by two major environmental features: the soft tissue environment and the bony base relationship (skeletal base relationship). The soft tissues comprise the lips, cheeks and tongue. The teeth erupt into a position of balance between these muscles, called the 'neutral zone'.

The bony base (*Fig. 6.4*) is an inherited feature upon which the alveolar processes are based. The alveolar processes contain the teeth and make up

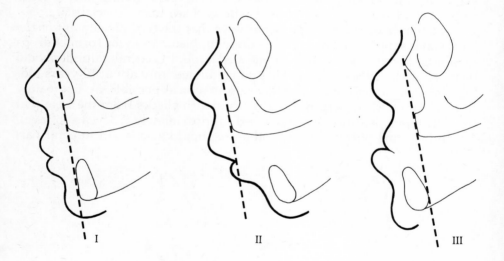

Fig. 6.4. Classification of skeletal relationship.

the dental arches. The class I skeletal base relationship is the relationship of the maxillary bony base where it lies slightly forwards of the mandibular bony base and is considered normal. In the skeletal II bony base relationship the mandibular bony base is significantly set back compared to the maxillary base. In the skeletal III bony base relationship the mandibular base may be too far forwards or the maxillary base may be set back or a combination of both.

In the cleft palate patient the child inherits the normal range of skeletal relationship; however, due to the cleft insult to the maxilla, this bony base is normally underdeveloped. Up to about 6 years old, the upper incisors normally remain in front of the lowers (class I) or tend to an edge to edge position (class III). The posterior segments will tend to have varying degrees of crossbite, with a number of upper posterior teeth biting inside the lowers. In the bilateral cleft the crossbite is seen bilaterally, whereas in the unilateral cleft the crossbite would be seen unilaterally. In this early phase, the minimum of orthodontic treatment should take place. Where there are misplaced deciduous teeth, which give rise to problems, such as a sore tongue from rubbing against a decayed edge, or a tooth preventing closure of a fistula, they will need to be removed. The earliest consideration for treatment

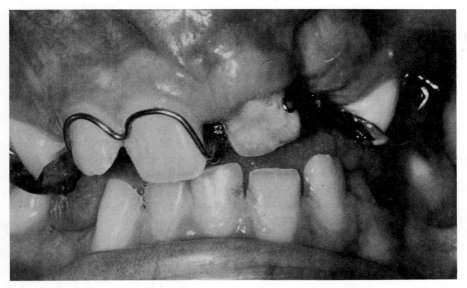

Fig. 6.5. An upper removable appliance with acrylic posterior bite planes used to open the incisor bite. A spring on the upper left incisor will procline the tooth.

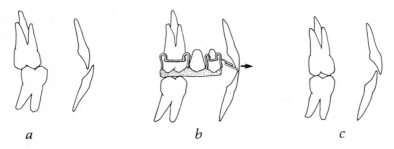

a *b* *c*

Fig. 6.6.*a.* Upper incisors behind lower incisions (class III) in displaced occlusion. *b.* Undisplaced incisor position with removable appliance. *c.* Normal corrected incisors (class I) stable position with positive overjet and overbite.

is usually the permanent upper incisors, when they erupt at about 6 years old (*Fig.* 6.6). Very often these teeth erupt behind the lower incisors. Usually this abnormal position will provoke a displacing movement of the lower jaw forwards, and this causes the permanent dentition to develop into an incorrect relationship. It is important to correct this displacing action. Simple removable appliances are used to move the upper incisors forwards and when this position is stable the dentition is left to continue its normal development with the eruption of the remainder of the permanent teeth.

MANAGEMENT IN THE PERMANENT DENTITION

The permanent dentition in the cleft lip and palate patient is affected in certain general ways:

1. The lateral incisor in the line of the cleft is missing or modified in size or shape.
2. The central incisor adjacent to the cleft is invariably poorly developed.
3. There are usually more missing teeth in cleft lip and palate patients than normal.
4. The permanent teeth are slower in erupting than the normal range.

The first phase of orthodontic treatment for the cleft patient is as described previously. The main aim will be to move the upper incisors forwards from behind the lower incisors. The severity of the cleft problem does not become fully apparent until puberty. At this time the restrictive effects on growth by scarring from earlier surgery has its greatest influence. Scarring across the midline narrows the arch and causes varying degrees of crossbite, with a number of upper posterior teeth biting inside the lowers. Scarring at the back of the upper arch will restrict the forward development of the maxilla. In addition, there is the normal spectrum of inherited jaw relationships, and so the range of effect for a cleft lip and palate patient may be quite wide. There can be minimal disturbance with a near normal incisor relationship, to quite severe reverse incisor positions, where even complex orthodontic treatment will not deal with the problem. A decision has to be made at this stage whether orthodontics alone will correct the problem, or whether a combination of orthodontics and surgery will be necessary to align the arches initially, and then surgically correct the bony base relationship.

Treatment will take place from 11 to 15 years of age, depending on individual dental development. In females puberty and dental development are usually two years in advance of males, and so will usually start that much earlier.

When gentle forces are applied to teeth they will move through bone. The bone resorbs on the pressure side and new bone is laid down by osteoblasts on the tension side. The simplest movements are produced by tipping forces. These forces may be applied by removable appliances with springs which move individual teeth in the required directions. In cleft lip and palate patients the first phase of treatment can be completed using removable appliances where the upper incisors are upright or retroclined and there is a displacing action present. Upper incisors with this angulation can be tipped forwards and they are likely to remain stable at the end of active treatment. The vertical overlap between upper and lower incisors will also encourage stability following this straightforward phase of active treatment.

In the final phase of orthodontic treatment for a cleft lip and palate patient, which may start at about age 11 years onwards, more complex movements are necessary. For these complex tooth movements such as derotation, uprighting, arch expansion and alignment, a fixed appliance is the orthodontic appliance of choice (*Fig.* 6.7). Individual bands or bonded brackets allow wires to be placed which will move the teeth precisely into the desired positions. There are a number of fixed appliance techniques and it is the choice of the operator as to which type of fixed appliance system is used. Treatment at this point is necessarily lengthy due to the extensive tooth movements required and will usually take about two years. The patient will attend an orthodontic clinic monthly for adjustments and changes. A mention should be made that tooth movements are not only made in a lateral or antero-posterior direction, but that there is also increasing evidence that vertical changes to the teeth may have significant beneficial effects on treatment of the cleft lip and palate patient.

Not all cleft lip and palate patients are suitable for complicated fixed appliances, and ultimately the same criteria as for any patient requiring orthodontics would need to be applied. These are basically that patient motivation must be high, hygiene must be good and also the quality of the teeth such that they would not be compromised during a lengthy fixed appliance treatment. There are some cases in the permanent dentition who would need only simple treatment to align anterior teeth, accepting a compromise in relation to crossbite. It is possible to replace missing incisor teeth and compensate for a posterior crossbite by using an overlay denture. The final most complicated group of cases where orthodontic correction alone is not possible — those who need fixed appliances prior to maxillo-facial surgery — will need extensive tooth movements to align both upper and lower arches. The aim in treatment of these cases is to get good alignment of both arches such that they will fit together precisely once the surgery is completed. There seems to be growing evidence that where there is good interlock between both arches following jaw surgery, then the occlusion remains stable (*see* Chapter 10).

Following orthodontic treatment it is necessary to hold the aligned teeth in their new positions. This allows the supporting bone to recover and the surrounding tissues such as lips, cheek and tongue, to readapt. A removable plastic plate is the most commonly used device. If there are missing teeth

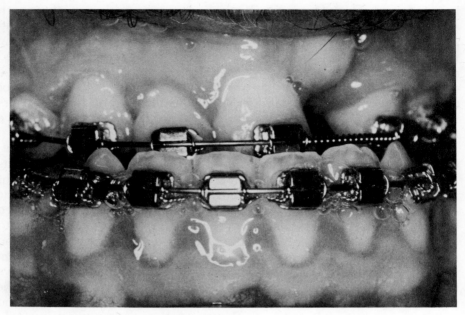

Fig. 6.7. A fixed appliance used to align upper and lower teeth prior to surgery.

this plate can include denture teeth. The nature of expansion in the upper arch, against scar tissue, is such that it is one of the most unstable tooth movements in orthodontics. To avoid relapse it is usually necessary to make two retainer appliances so that if one is broken another can be placed immediately. It is of considerable importance that when a patient goes for secondary plastic surgery or maxillo-facial correction that the retainers are replaced immediately after the surgery where this is appropriate. In the unstable situation, two years of hard work may be undone within a matter of days if such retention appliances are left out. Careful counselling of the ward staff is necessary to prevent such disasters. Often the appliances will be worn for a number of years continuing into the late teens. It will then be possible to consider whether fixed retention with a bridge or continued removable appliance retention is needed. At this later stage patients with a severe bony base problem (*Fig.* 6.8) will need to have their maxillo-facial jaw surgery carried out. The treatment is planned between the oral surgeon, plastic surgeon and the orthodontist to achieve the best possible results.

It is important during the treatment of cleft lip and palate patients to take good records, the orthodontist being in the best position to do this. At the very least they should include study model impressions taken at key times during development and lateral skull X-rays taken at similar times to the study model impressions. This combination of tooth and skeletal information allows retrospective studies of changes taking place during orthodontics and general growth considerations.

A technique which has an increasing role to play is bone grafting. This will take place at the age when the permanent upper canines have two-thirds root development, and this can be from age 9 years onwards, depending on individual dental development. Missing alveolar bone in the region of the cleft can be replaced by inserting bone chips taken from the

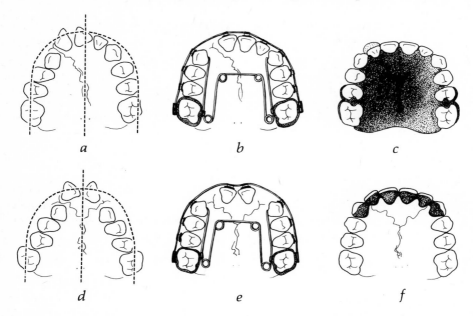

Fig. 6.8.*a.* Missing upper right lateral incisors. Collapse of upper right segment giving rise to 'cross-bite'. *b.* Expansion of upper right segment, with fixed appliance. *c.* Retention holding the arch alignment with a simple denture replacing the upper right lateral incisor. *d.* Missing upper lateral incisors. Collapse of left and right segments — bilateral 'cross-bite'. *e.* Expansion of upper posterior segments with fixed appliance. *f.* Retention and replacement of upper lateral incisors by fixed bridgework.

hip or ribs. This will help establish a more normal arch form which will support the nose and provide a field for eruption of the canines. Bone grafting can reduce the need for replacement of missing incisors by dental appliances, encouraging a more normal contact between the canines and incisors. Its application is likely to become increasingly important in the future. Finally, it must always be borne in mind that every patient has a limited level of tolerance. Treatment should therefore be kept as simple as possible and should not involve too many active stages.

Chapter 7

Type and assessment of speech problems

E.H. Albery

The ability to communicate effectively with others is vital if we are to function as accepted members of our society. For normal speech we need adequate hearing and the ability to interpret speech and form concepts, which may then be expressed as words via the vocal tract.

What Is 'Cleft Palate' Speech?
The vocal tract consists of the lungs, larynx, pharynx, oral and nasal cavities, hard and soft palates, the tongue, teeth and lips. Cleft palate is classed in speech terms as a 'structural disorder' of this tract. Children with repaired cleft palates often have difficulties with the expression of speech, which are not like those difficulties experienced by other groups of speech-impaired children. It is easier to understand why 'cleft palate' speech occurs if we view the vocal tract as a system dependent upon correctly regulated air pressure (*Fig. 7.1*).

In English there are 23 consonants, 15 vowel sounds and nine diphthongs. For 'normal' speech to occur, air is pumped from the lungs and passes through the larynx where, if the vocal folds are together and vibrating, a 'voiced' sound is heard, e.g. 'b', 'v'; if the vocal folds are apart a 'voiceless' sound is heard, e.g. 'p', 'f'. Almost simultaneously air enters the oral cavity which, for all sounds except 'm', 'n', 'ng' is separated from the nasal cavity by the upward and backward movement of the soft palate, forward movement of the posterior pharyngeal wall and inward movement of the lateral pharyngeal walls (*Fig. 7.2*). The air is then modified by the movements of the tongue and lips to form different consonant and vowel sounds.

It is usual for a cleft palate to be repaired before two years of age, but, if a cleft involving the soft palate has not been repaired or the soft palate is not functioning adequately after repair, an effective seal cannot be made

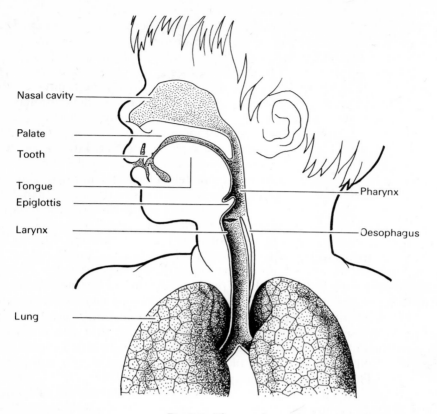

Nasal cavity

Palate

Tooth

Tongue

Epiglottis

Larynx

Lung

Pharynx

Oesophagus

Fig. 7.1. The vocal tract.

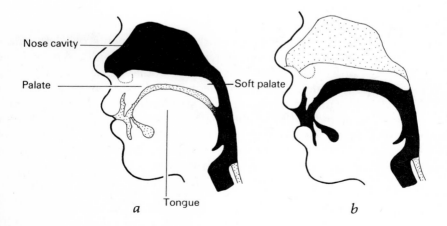

Nose cavity

Palate

Soft palate

a   Tongue

b

Fig. 7.2. *a*. Soft palate at rest (breathing). *b*. Soft palate during speech.

between the oral and nasal cavities and air will escape during speech. This will have the direct effect of producing more or less audible nasal escape of air accompanying pressure consonant sounds, such as 'p', 'b', 't', 'd', 's', 'z', usually in conjunction with an excessive nasal tone heard on vowel sounds, which is known as hypernasality. Normal functioning of the velopharyngeal sphincter is also critical for the correct development of consonant and vowel sounds, commonly known as 'articulation'. Generally, the worse the degree of velopharyngeal incompetence, the worse affected is the articulation. However, despite gross velopharyngeal incompetence, some children manage to develop normal articulation while others, even with an early successful palate repair, develop very deviant articulation. The most popular theory as to the cause of much of the deviant articulation in cleft palate speakers is that the disturbance in the air pressure balance of the vocal tract leads indirectly to deviant tongue movements or inappropriate constrictions of the glottis or pharynx (see Fig. 7.1), in an effort to compensate for lack of adequate intra-oral air pressure.

It seems that these compensations begin during the first year of life, generally before the palate has been repaired. An infant begins to produce syllables which are rapidly modelled on the sounds he hears other people make. His attempts at these sounds, for which he will almost certainly lack sufficient intra-oral air pressure before palate repair, and also a normal configuration of the hard and soft palates for the tongue to articulate against, may well result in the setting up of compensatory movements within the vocal tract. These movements may become habitual.

The cleft palate infant may also have fluid within the middle ear which will have a dampening effect on his hearing and thus his ability to imitate sounds accurately. Indeed, throughout childhood the cleft palate child is very likely to have a fluctuating conductive hearing loss which, if severe enough, will affect his speech.

Functional Versus Organic Disorders

It is important to distinguish between those components of 'cleft palate speech' which are *organic* and those which are *functional* . An example of an *organic* disorder is consistent nasal escape and hypernasality following cleft palate repair, which point to inadequate velopharyngeal closure. A *functional* disorder may originate from a structural disorder, e.g. deviant articulation associated with the cleft palate, or inconsistent nasal escape and hypernasality. As a very general rule, organic disorders of velopharyngeal function should be treated surgically, whilst functional disorders should be treated with speech therapy.

THE ASSESSMENT OF CLEFT PALATE SPEECH

When a speech therapist assesses the speech of a child with a cleft palate or a related velopharyngeal problem, he or she needs to separate three broad

aspects of cleft palate speech:
1. Nasal escape.
2. Nasal resonance.
3. Articulation.

The first two are indicative of velopharyngeal sufficiency or insufficiency, which is the most difficult area for speech therapists to assess, particularly if they are not very familiar with the speech problems of cleft palate children. Notwithstanding, it is of vital importance that an organic velopharyngeal incompetence should be recognized as soon as possible and referred to a plastic surgeon for investigation and surgery. The days should be long past when a speech therapist and her 'charge' were expected to struggle for years to try and overcome an organic velopharyngeal insufficiency.

Assessment of Nasal Escape

For most speech therapists, the assessment of nasal escape is a subjective judgement due to the cost of equipment for detecting nasal escape. A nasal anemometer, for example, has been developed in Exeter and is an extremely useful machine to indicate when and approximately how much nasal escape is occurring during speech. If a nasal anemometer is not available, the therapist should at least attempt to grade the nasal escape she hears. A four point scale should be adequate for most purposes, i.e. slight, moderate, gross, variable. Variable nasal escape, for example only occurring on 's' and 'z', denotes a functional disorder and should be treated accordingly. The degree of audible nasal escape correlates quite highly with the size of the velopharyngeal gap. Therefore, in many cases, an estimate may be made by the therapist as to the degree of velopharyngeal insufficiency. Care must be taken, however, when assessing nasal escape and hence estimating the size of velopharyngeal gap in certain groups of patients. Examples are patients with a 'glottal stop' pattern of articulation who constrict the air stream at the level of the glottis and thus very little air diffuses into the nasal cavity to be perceived as nasal escape. If the same patient is taught to articulate correctly, more nasal escape may become evident and, in such a case, the size of the velopharyngeal gap is probably bigger than was at first predicted. However, one should always be aware of the possibility of *potential* competence and, if a patient is exhibiting a total glottal stop pattern, he or she may not be using the palate to its full potential. A short period of diagnostic therapy is, therefore, indicated so that at least one or two consonants are produced correctly without glottalization ('p' or 'b' for example). Together with investigations undertaken by a plastic surgeon, potential movement of the velopharyngeal isthmus can then be assessed. Other examples of difficulty in assessing the degree of velopharyngeal insufficiency include the presence of a cold, which may prevent or change the perception of nasal escape, a deviated nasal septum, a nostril stenosis, an aspirate voice, or simply talking very quietly so that it is difficult to hear the nasal escape. A hard palate fistula, which is more common than one in the soft palate, may be responsible for some nasal escape of air, so that, when assessing velopharyngeal insufficiency, it is advisable to block the fistula temporarily with dental wax, or chewing gum.

Nasal Resonance

In a case of velopharyngeal insufficiency the degree of hypernasality or excessive nasal resonance, usually correlates with the degree of nasal escape. The therapist again has to rely on subjective judgement in assessing nasal resonance. It is important for the clinician who is inexperienced in listening to cleft palate speech to learn to differentiate between hypernasality (excessive nasal resonance) and hyponasality (insufficient nasal resonance). A reasonable sample of spontaneous speech should be obtained on which to base one's judgement of perceived hypernasality and it is useful to ask a child of the appropriate age, from five years onwards, to count to 20 so that one can attempt to rate the nasal resonance. The nasal resonance can then be graded:

Normal	0	Slight hyponasality	−1
Slight hypernasality	1	Moderate hyponasality	−2
Moderate hypernasality	2	Gross hyponasality	−3
Gross hypernasality	3	Mixed resonance	4

Causes of Hyponasality

Hyponasality is generally more acceptable to our ear than is hypernasality, but, if severe enough, it can certainly make speech sound unacceptable. We all sound hyponasal or denasal when we have a cold (in fact, the opposite of sounding 'nasal'). Hyponasality can also occur due to any blocking of the resonating chambers. Some common disorders which cause hyponasality are enlarged adenoids, the presence of polyps, or blocked sinuses, or it may occur following a pharyngoplasty.

Assessment of Articulation

It is necessary to assess three 'levels' of articulation in order that appropriate management may be planned: consonants in isolation, in single words and in continuous speech.

Consonants in isolation. It is useful for the cleft palate child or adult to imitate the therapist in producing all consonants in isolation. Sometimes the production of consonants in isolation is better than their production in continuous speech but more often the difficulties the patient is experiencing in speaking are highlighted by his attempts at isolated consonants. This indicates the level at which therapy should commence.

Single words. There are various articulation tests which a speech therapist can utilize for single word testing. In the United States, one of the most widely used is the Iowa Pressure Articulation Test (IPAT). One possible criticism of tests such as the IPAT, which are aimed specifically at identifying 'cleft palate' errors, is that they do not give complete information. Thus, it is useful to ensure that one obtains a sample of each consonant, and not selected consonants, as it occurs initially and finally in words, and that a reasonable sample of consonant clusters is heard. Large photographs of familiar everyday things can be organized to cover all consonants and these can be shown to children aged between three and ten years. Older children can read out a word list.

Continuous speech. A reasonable sample (1-2 minutes) of spontaneous speech should be obtained. For younger children (18 months to 4 years old), this sample can be obtained through play, or the reciting of nursery rhymes. Speech may deteriorate markedly when it is spontaneous, as opposed to when a child is making every effort to produce correct consonants. Even 'spontaneous' speech in the clinic may not represent a true picture of a child's performance. The acid test of spontaneous speech would be to hear a child chatting to friends in the school playground.

A high quality cassette recorder is recommended to record each assessment so that the recording may be played back to aid accurate transcription of the utterance.

Physical Examination
A routine oral examination should be performed, to provide information on the possible relevance to speech of abnormalities of the lips, teeth, alveolar arch, hard and soft palates and tongue. It is unusual these days for an upper lip to be so short and/or immobile that speech is affected. Teeth may be missing, or misaligned, and may affect consonant production; the alveolar arch may be collapsed and narrow; the presence of a fistula in either the hard or soft palates should be noted. Occasionally this may affect articulation as the patient tries to cover the 'hole' with his tongue during speech, but nasal escape is more often attributable to a velopharyngeal problem than to a hard palate fistula. It is unusual for tongue movement itself to be a problem, although deviant patterns may be observed during speech.

A marked malocclusion may predispose the child or adult to difficulties, with sibilant sounds, such as 's' and 'z'.

Finally, it should be emphasized that many children are able to compensate for slight or moderate degrees of structural abnormality as far as their articulation is concerned. Some children with missing teeth, a collapsed alveolar arch and a class III angle malocclusion may produce acoustically normal speech, whilst other children with only very slight structural abnormalities have much more difficulty in producing acceptable speech. With all articulatory disorders, account has to be taken of factors such as hearing acuity, auditory discrimination and self-monitoring skills, motivation, intelligence and family background.

Chapter 8

The management of cleft palate speech

E.H. Albery

The timing of the initial assessment of speech and language in cleft palate children varies among speech therapists as does the timing of intervention. A therapist working in a Regional Plastic Surgery Unit has the opportunity of meeting cleft palate babies and their families before the babies are a year old and may instigate programmes to prevent language delay, or to identify and correct deviant articulation, like the so-called 'glottal babbling' before the toddler has reached his second birthday. Some speech therapists may recommend secondary surgery for speech in the form of a pharyngoplasty (*see* Chapter 5) below three years of age. Probably around 50 per cent of cleft palate children develop acceptable articulation on their own and 70-90 per cent do not need further surgery for velopharyngeal insufficiency. Therefore, a balance has to be achieved on the one hand between not rushing into therapy or surgery unnecessarily and, on the other, not leaving speech, language or surgical intervention so late that a child suffers socially and emotionally because of his/her speech.

The Pre-school Child
About the earliest one can generally obtain a reasonable sample of speech on which to base an assessment of articulation and velopharyngeal sufficiency, is age two to three years. Following assessment, various decisions can be made as to further management depending on the individual speech problems.

Articulation
Regarding problems of *articulation* in two to three year olds, the following categories provide a very simple guide to management:

1. *No action: review around school age*
   Cleft palate children with normal articulation appropriate to their age.

2. *Three-monthly review*
   Children who have deviant articulation, but are showing signs that it is becoming normal. These children should be watched to check that their speech continues to develop towards the normal.

3. *Regular speech therapy*
   Children who show a significant delay in expressive speech which can occur with or without articulatory deviances associated with the cleft palate, or who demonstrate deviant 'cleft palate' type speech alone. On the whole, the more intensive the therapy, the more quickly results will be achieved, but where this is impractical and the child has a supportive and caring family, once-weekly therapy, backed up with daily practice at home, may achieve good results.

Velopharyngeal Insufficiency
The significance of the identification of velopharyngeal insufficiency between two and three years of age is variable.

1. *Slight incompetence with slight nasal escape and hypernasality*
   This level of velopharyngeal insufficiency may sometimes resolve spontaneously by school age as the child becomes more self-conscious and learns to compensate.

2. *Moderate or gross velopharyngeal insufficiency and very deviant articulation*
   A therapist may try a short period of diagnostic therapy to see if the insufficiency and/or deviant articulation will improve, but if they don't, then surgery, followed by speech therapy, is likely to be the management procedure of choice.

3. *Moderate or gross velopharyngeal insufficiency with good articulation*
   A child may need surgery alone to effect a dramatic improvement in speech. Hypernasality is an ugly voice quality and, although good articulation is more crucial for intelligibility than nasality, children are teased just as much about 'talking down their nose' as about poor consonant production.

4. *Variable velopharyngeal sufficiency*
   Children who articulate one or two consonant sounds (usually 's' and 'z') nasally, and who have no significant nasal escape on other 'pressure' sounds, e.g. 'p', 'b', 't', 'd', should be treated with speech

therapy, not surgery. A pharyngoplasty would serve only to reduce the velopharyngeal isthmus and risk making all the speech hyponasal. Speech therapy should teach the child a new habit of directing air orally on 's' and 'z'. This phenomenon has been described as the 'discouraged' 's' or a palate 'rhythm' fault.

It is evident when working with cleft palate children, as with any other speech-impaired children, that each individual's management programme has to be tailored to meet his/her specific needs. This is exemplified in cases of 'borderline' velopharyngeal sufficiency, when perhaps there is slight audible nasal escape and hypernasality throughout speech despite a period of speech therapy. One family may find this degree of impairment unacceptable and request surgery for their child. Another family may not even be aware of the same level of impairment in their own child and, therefore, surgery probably would not be appropriate for that child at that time. Of course, he or she may reach adolescence and become aware and self-conscious about speech and may then request surgery.

The School Child

Ideally, children with a cleft palate should have achieved good enough speech not to draw comment from their peers by the time they are starting school, but this is not always possible. Reasons may include inadequate density of therapy pre-school, an unsupportive family background where the importance of good speech is not recognized, lack of cooperation and motivation in therapy sessions, low IQ or frequent occurrence of hearing loss due to the fluctuating conductive deafness commonly found in cleft palate children.

In addition, the surgical assessment of velopharyngeal insufficiency (by radiology and nasal pharyngoscopy) is easier the older the child, particularly with regard to endoscopy. If, in the pre-school years, there is evidence of velopharyngeal insufficiency, but this does not appear to be having a significant effect on consonant production, it may be wise to wait until a child has started school before investigations take place, as they are more likely to be successful and give the surgeon the best possible information on which to base his operation. If, however, there is gross velopharyngeal insufficiency which seems to prevent articulation development, surgery may be indicated for children of three to five years old even without investigation. Following successful surgery, in the experience of most clinicians, speech therapy usually produces more rapid improvement in articulation. Speech therapy may well continue into the school years, either at the hospital where the cleft palate was repaired, the local health clinic or at the child's school where a speech therapist may work one or two sessions a week. A proportion of children who do not make progress with conventional weekly therapy require more intensive help and residential courses of therapy are available in a few regional hospitals around the country.

Adult

There is no age limit for 'normal' speech to be achieved. Cleft palate adults in their forties and fifties who have presented at clinics, not having been followed up since the initial palate repair, have undergone a successful pharyngoplasty to cure velopharyngeal insufficiency and a course of speech therapy to improve articulation. Provided the patient is motivated to improve his/her speech, the correct production of consonants in isolation and, their generalization into everyday speech, can be achieved.

TYPE OF THERAPY

Therapy for Nasality

It is obvious from the preceding pages that a consistent, moderate degree of velopharyngeal insufficiency, which is not improved significantly by a short period of speech therapy, should be treated surgically. In a few cases (usually where glottal stops replace all pressure consonant sounds), improvement in articulation automatically triggers the palate to move appropriately, so a period of diagnostic therapy before committing a child or adult to surgery is wise. Inconsistent velopharyngeal insufficiency should be treated with speech therapy unless it is caused by a severe sensori-neural deafness, when improvement may well be very difficult to achieve. A technique which should produce success with children who direct the airstream nasally rather than orally for 's' and 'z' is to work from a pressure consonant they can produce orally, for example /t/, and ask them to prolong the sound. Alternatively one can ask them to move their tongue forward from a 'S' (pronounced 'sh') or backwards from a 'θ' (pronounced 'th'). As long as the child doesn't realize in the first instance that they are being asked to produce an 's', and it just 'happens' using one of the above techniques, very rapid progress can usually be made.

Feedback Devices

Where there is evidence of inappropriate timing in movement of the soft palate, or nasal escape due to lack of palate mobility, the Selley palatal training appliance and visual speech aid may be useful and, in the latter case, may avoid the need for surgery. A nasal anemometer which allows the presence of nasal escape to be displayed on a meter can be used to show a patient what happens when he lifts his palate. This is an example of visual feedback. For auditory feedback, a tape recording and playback of a patient's speech can be helpful. Slight or variable degrees of hypernasality and nasal escape may be controlled in this way, although reduction of nasality in single words alone is not enough and therapy should be continued until control of nasal escape is possible in continuous speech.

Therapy for Articulation

In this writer's experience, conventional articulation therapy has produced improvement in articulation for the vast majority of children treated, and is always used as a 'first line' approach with the addition of other approaches from time to time.

Having identified the deviant consonants, articulation therapy can be planned. This type of therapy consists of five 'stages':

1. The correct production of consonants in isolation.
2. Consonant plus vowel combinations.
3. Single words.
4. Sentences.
5. Everyday speech.

It appears that stages 1 and 5, which are the most difficult to achieve, are the stages most helped by intensive therapy. Unlike children who have a phonological speech problem, the speech problems of cleft palate children are usually at the basic level of consonants in isolation because of the original structural disorder, and are usually consistent throughout speech. A technique often has to be found to show a child how to produce a 't' or an 's' and, once achieved, to progress through the various stages. Where the production of a consonant in isolation, for example 't', is proving difficult, proprioception neuromuscular facilitation techniques (PNF), e.g. contrasting heat with cold on the tongue tip as it comes into contact with the alveolar ridge, or a dental plate with a ridge made where the tongue should touch for 't' (or possibly myofunctional therapy), may solve the problem. Often the cleft palate children exhibit a number of consonants with the same deviant feature, e.g. glottalization, palatalization or velarization. It is useful to tackle as many of the deviant consonant sounds as possible at the same time so a new 'pattern' is quickly established.

Blowing and Sucking

Although the evidence for blowing and sucking exercises in improving velopharyngeal function is lacking, where an improvement in oral breath direction for consonant production is required, e.g. with glottal stop articulation, gentle blowing with phonation can help to provide this initially, the blowing element gradually being phased out and a consonant such as 'p' introduced with the phonation.

CONCLUSION

Of utmost importance is the recognition of velopharyngeal insufficiency which requires surgery. Then, a speech therapist has to be able to deal with any articulation problems with an adequate density of speech therapy for the problem and appropriate techniques of therapy to tackle the sometimes very deviant speech which can still be observed in this group of children. Provided these criteria are fulfilled, the vast majority of cleft palate children will enjoy the ability to communicate effectively, perhaps the most important goal in their overall management.

Chapter 9

Ear disease

A. Richard Maw

For many years it had been appreciated that there was a significant relationship between the presence of a cleft palate and ear disease in children and subsequently in later life. A detectable hearing loss or the presence of abnormalities of the eardrum was, therefore, expected in children with cleft palate and, depending upon which aspect was studied, as many as half or three-quarters of individuals were found to be affected in this way.

However, more recently, careful examination with an otoscope to view the ear drum in children before palatal repair has been performed, confirms that there is a middle ear effusion in almost all such children under two years of age. These effusions are collections of fluid within the middle ear (*Fig.* 9.1) which may be either serous (thin) or mucoid (thick) and frequently the latter is referred to as 'glue ear'. The incidence of these effusions decreases significantly once the cleft palate has been repaired.

It is for these reasons that, in many departments dealing with cleft palates, children are routinely referred to an ear, nose and throat surgeon (ENT surgeon) for examination of their ears. This may be arranged before the palate is repaired or afterwards and will provide an opportunity to explain the association between the disorder and the middle ear and hearing problems. Thus forewarned, the parents should be less alarmed than they might otherwise have been when the first episode of otitis media develops. They will also be alert to the other manifestations and they should now have in their ENT surgeon an ally whose help they can seek should simple measures fail to relieve their problems. Follow-up appointments will be continued until the surgeon is satisfied that the condition of the ears is acceptable and the hearing ability is within normal limits.

There is now evidence to confirm that the middle ear problems, and in particular the accumulation of fluid in the middle ear, results from improper functioning of the eustachian tube. It fails to open normally during

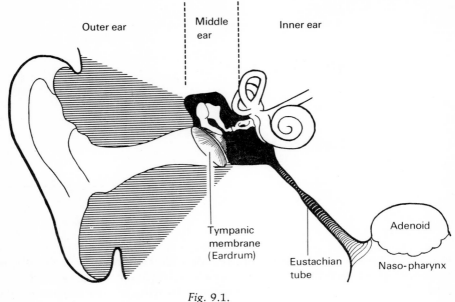

Fig. 9.1.

swallowing and a negative pressure develops within the middle ear space. This pressure can now be detected very simply by impedance audiometry, which has become a standard procedure in most clinics. A soft probe is inserted into the ear canal and a sound stimulus is presented. By altering the pressure within the ear canal it is possible to measure the stiffness of the ear drum and middle ear mechanism and also to measure the middle ear pressure. The procedure is painless and does not require very much cooperation from the child, so is available for use in smaller children. Although the eustachian tube is anatomically patent there is a functional blockage due to malfunction of the opening mechanism caused by displacement of the tensor and levator palati muscles due to the cleft in the palate. Following repair of the cleft the eustachian tube function improves and middle ear complications diminish. Unfortunately, the underlying disorder is not always totally correctable and as a result these children are more susceptible to chronic malfunction of their eustachian tubes. In addition to this there is frequently an inflammatory process which usually presents as a middle ear infection.

Other factors may affect eustachian tube function, such as an alteration in the shape of the facial or skull bones or an enlargement or infection of the adenoids in the roof of the nasopharynx. In children with nasal and sinus disease the presence within the nasopharynx of infected material may predispose to ascending eustachian tube infection. Similarly, any generalized abnormality of the respiratory tract mucous membrane may lead to eustachian tube malfunction. This may occur with any bacterial or viral infection or as a result of allergy or may result from the effect of irritants, such as chlorinated swimming pool water.

It is thus apparent that almost all the middle ear problems which arise in association with cleft palate are related indirectly to the eustachian tube. As a result a conductive hearing loss develops. There is poor conduction of the sound pressure wave through the middle ear space due to the accumulation of fluid or infected material — in a few cases a sensori-neural hearing loss may develop from extension of the inflammatory process from the middle ear into the inner ear, but this is uncommon. The two types of hearing loss can be distinguished by clinical examination together with pure tone audiometry and impedance audiometry.

CLINICAL FEATURES

The clinical features which result from the middle ear changes vary according to the age of the patient and the severity of the disease. In infants and smaller children there may be clearcut signs, such as discharge from the ear, or the condition may be less obvious. The child may pull at the ear, often causing abrasions. There may be irritability, fever, screaming attacks or sleep disturbance. In older children, earache may become a frequent occurrence and is often followed by discharge from the ear. However, the changes may be more insidious resulting from undetected hearing loss. Thus speech development may be delayed, language and communication impeded and subtle effects on emotional, intellectual and learning processes may arise. In five-year-olds, an unsuspected hearing loss can present at school as difficulty or delay in reading and often it is the teacher, an outsider or grandparent who suspects the loss rather than the child's parents for whom the condition has become accepted. The increased volume of the television, a tendency to shout and behavioural difficulties are frequently seen as part of the normal process of 'growing up' and this is particularly so if there are co-existent and more obviously distressing problems such as a cleft palate or cleft lip.

The diagnosis of otitis media is easier in older children and teenagers particularly if there is discharge, pain, a sense of blockage, disturbance of balance or tinnitus. Regardless of age there is always the possibility of more serious complications developing. A spread of infection from the ear to the meninges can give rise to meningitis and other intra-cranial problems but happily nowadays these are uncommon.

MANAGEMENT

Assessment of the middle ear in very young babies is difficult. Wax must be gently removed from the ear canal before examination of the eardrum can be made with an otoscope. Movement of the eardrum can be assessed by attachment of a small pneumatic bulb to the otoscope. In older children hearing ability for pure tone sounds is assessed by audiometry and the middle

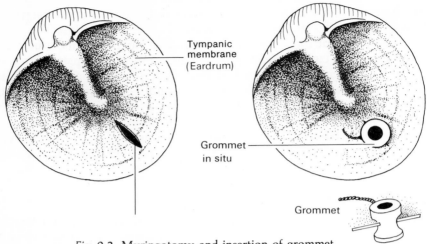

Tympanic membrane (Eardrum)

Grommet in situ

Grommet

Fig. 9.2. Myringotomy and insertion of grommet.

ear mechanism and middle ear pressure is investigated by an impedance audiometer. Usually a regular follow-up appointment will be made and the child's condition will be reviewed until the ENT surgeon is satisfied that the ears and hearing ability are within acceptable limits. Often parents will not be aware of any problems with their child's ears and, despite this, the surgeon may find a middle ear effusion on examination. He will continue to review the child until either the effusion resolves spontaneously or it is decided that treatment is required.

Episodes of acute infection presenting with pain may respond to medication with simple pain relievers such as aspirin. For more severe infections where often discharge is present, antibiotics may be required. Sometimes these may be prescribed for longer periods than is usual. Decongestants may be used to improve more generalized catarrh and sometimes nose drops are helpful.

The hearing loss which results from a long-standing middle ear effusion usually requires surgical treatment. The fluid can be drained from the middle ear by myringotomy. This will require general anaesthesia but can be easily arranged on a day care basis. Unfortunately, the effect is often short-lived and reaccumulation of the middle ear fluid which follows myringotomy alone has led to the introduction of grommets. These are small plastic or Teflon tubes with a lumen; they can be placed through the incision in the eardrum to provide ventilation. Provided the lumen remains patent the effusion does not usually recur. However, there are a certain number of cases in which there is discharge through the lumen of the grommet and sometimes this requires treatment with eardrops and antibiotics before it resolves. The grommets remain in place for varying periods of time and may last for 12 to 15 months. Usually, however, they are extruded spontaneously within 6 months. If middle ear fluid reaccumulates and is accompanied by a significant hearing loss, a grommet may need to be re-inserted (*Fig.* 9.2).

If there is evidence of nasal or sinus disease, a sinus washout can be performed under the same anaesthetic. Adenoidectomy may be recommended if the adenoids are thought to be affecting eustachian tube function either as a result of their size or their persistent infection. Only in exceptional circumstances, such as very frequent episodes of tonsillitis, is tonsillectomy advised.

The child with a cleft palate will become a regular attender at an ear, nose and throat clinic and, unfortunately, the complications which may arise as a result of the middle ear disease, will lead to their subsequent attendance in these clinics during adulthood.

Chapter 10

Oral surgery

G. Pell

INTRODUCTION

Any reconstructive oral surgery for the cleft palate patient is carried out
when maxillary growth has ceased. Until this stage has been reached, oral
surgery is limited to surgical orthodontic problems, which are likely to
impede the orthodontic treatment which is proposed, e.g. removal of
supernumerary teeth or misplaced canines. Throughout the growing period,
however, the patient is regularly examined at a joint clinic until the correct
time for surgery has been reached, which is usually from the late teens
onwards.

ORAL SURGICAL PROBLEMS

The bony deformities seen in the cleft palate patient not only involve the
maxilla, but can also secondarily involve the mandible.

The main defects in the mid-facial bones are as follows:

    A The bony clefts:
        1. Unilateral clefts.
        2. Bilateral clefts.

    B A disturbance in directional growth:
        1. A horizontal direction (antero-posterior and lateral).
        2. A vertical direction.
        3. Both horizontal and vertical directions — the most usual.

The defect in the mandible appears as a real or an apparent prognathism
which may be accentuated by the lack of mid-facial bony growth, with
the result that the patient's occlusion and profile is markedly skeletal III

(*see* Chapter 6).

The aim of oral surgical treatment is to correct:

 a. The antero-posterior and lateral bony discrepancies.
 b. The vertical bony discrepancy of the maxilla (and the mandible where necessary).

By correcting the bony relationship surgically it will be possible to establish a good dental occlusion. This is achieved by performing an osteotomy on the facial skeleton and repositioning the mobilized bony blocks of mandible and maxilla into predetermined positions, relative to each other, so that the occlusion and facial appearance of the patient is both functionally and aesthetically improved.

PRE-SURGICAL MANAGEMENT

Prior to oral surgery being carried out on the cleft lip and palate patient, ideally there should be a careful and coordinated review programme arranged through the joint clinic, so that an assessment is made by all the disciplines in the team at the same time. This usually involves regular reviews until bony growth has ceased. By this time orthodontics may well have been completed, and the patient is wearing retainer appliances, or the orthodontic appliances are still being worn and can be included in the surgical treatment to be planned.

From an oral surgical point of view a diagnosis must be made in order to determine the extent of the maxillary and mandibular abnormalities, and also to assess how much the bony blocks need to be repositioned in both vertical and horizontal directions.

In order to achieve this, a number of investigations are carried out, which may include:

1. Accurate and up-to-date articulated dental study models.
2. A standard right lateral skull cephalogram in occlusion, taken at six feet.
3. An orthopantomogram.
4. A right lateral black and white photograph taken with the patient in occlusion at six feet.
5. A standard set of colour slides.

A number of life-sized photographic prints of the patient's right profile are prepared on clear acetate paper by the photographic department before treatment planning can be started. By superimposing the acetate print onto the lateral skull X-ray, various cephalometric bony landmarks and points are traced onto the print. By tracing the outline of the facial skeleton and teeth onto the acetate paper (*Fig.* 10.1*a*), a composite picture is built up of soft tissues, bony and dental points. An assessment of the cephalometric points, lines and angles will determine where the bony abnormality in the skeleton lies, and any directional deficiency will become apparent.

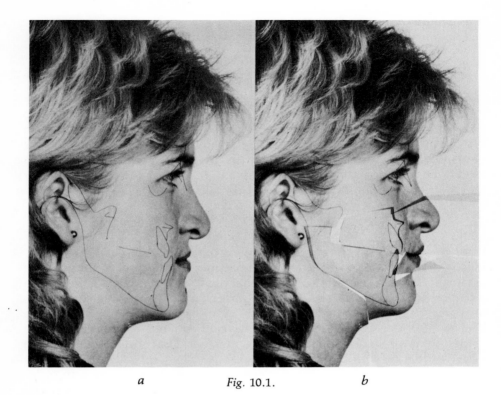

a   *Fig.* 10.1.   *b*

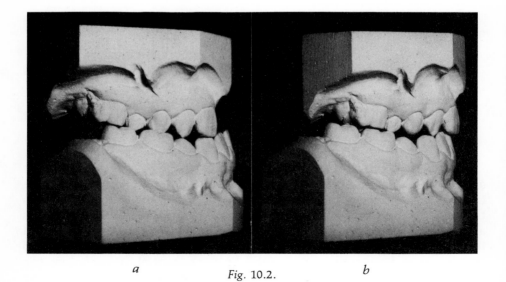

a   *Fig.* 10.2.   *b*

The study models (*Fig. 10.2a*) are manipulated in an antero-posterior direction until the best possible occlusion is obtained (*Fig. 10.2b*). It may be necessary to section two study models in order to align the various maxillary segments in such a way as to simulate the surgical procedure.

The acetate photograph is now sectioned in the planned way (*Fig. 10.1b*) together with the soft tissues so that the occlusion on the photograph is similar to the occlusion obtained on the study models. The photographic changes will determine by how much the various bony parts need to be moved in order to achieve as near normal a soft tissue and skeletal profile as possible.

Having determined these facts, and discussed them with the patient, an important step is to allow the patient to discuss the operation with a cleft lip and palate patient who has already undergone a similar procedure. The patient must also be warned that rib bone grafts may be needed and fixation of the jaws will be from 8 to 10 weeks.

Before the operation, cast silver splints are constructed and these should occlude accurately and easily with the planned post-operative jaw position, as determined from the study models and acetate photographs. This will provide the guide for the correct antero-posterior, lateral and vertical changes which have previously been assessed.

THE SURGICAL OPERATION

Before the operation the splints are cemented into the teeth. The planned procedure may involve either one jaw only, or both maxilla and mandible and, in the latter case, both jaws are corrected at the same operation.

The maxilla may be sectioned from the facial skeleton at various levels depending on the planned needs, but the most common site is at the Le Fort I level (*Fig. 10.3*).

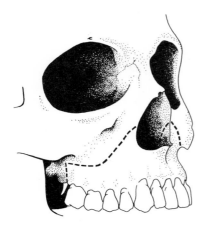

Fig. 10.3. The Le Fort I cut.

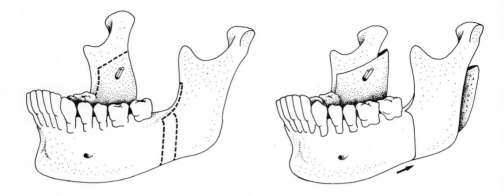

Fig. 10.4. Sagittal split mandibular osteotomy.

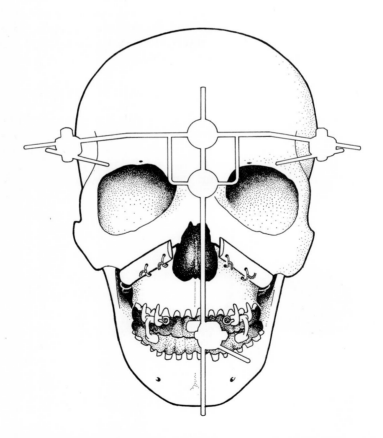

Fig. 10.5. Cranio-maxillary external fixation showing cast silver cap splints and bone grafts.

After reflecting the oral muco-periosteum from one maxillary tuberosity to the other, and dissecting into the tissues around the cleft, bilateral burr cuts are made in the bone of the lateral nasal wall on each side, through the maxillary bone to the posterior parts of the maxilla ending at the pterygo-maxillary fissures. The nasal septum is separated from the nasal surface of the hard palate and the pterygoid plates detached from the posterior part of the maxilla with an osteotome.

Scarring in the cleft and pterygoid regions may hinder manipulation and advancement of the maxillary segments, but, with care and determination, the segments will become mobile and advancement achieved.

If the cleft deformity is such that a mandibular procedure is also necessary, this osteotomy is performed at the same time and the predetermined occlusion is established.

A variety of osteotomies have been documented, but the intra-oral sagittal split procedure, with or without a sliding genioplasty, is commonly used. This involves bilaterally sectioning the rami of the mandible in the sagittal plane through the cancellous bone using burrs and osteotomes and repositioning the mobile fragment of the mandible into its new position, in relation to the mobilized maxilla (*Fig.* 10.4). At the same time, the chin point can be detached and repositioned as predetermined at the acetate planning stage.

Before immobilizing the facial bony fragments, the facial height may require elongating in the mid-facial region. This is achieved by elongating the maxillary/mandibular block at the Le Fort I level through the external fixation. The gap thus created at the Le Fort I bone cut is grafted with split rib bone which has been softened to the consistency of wet cardboard, and then wired across the maxillary defect. The bone is also carefully placed into the cleft space and the whole system then bolted and immobilized with external cranio-maxillary fixation (*Fig.* 10.5). Alternative methods of fixation may be employed, for example internal fixation using wires or plates.

POST-SURGICAL MANAGEMENT

The patients' jaws are immobilized by the cranio-facial fixation for 8-10 weeks and, during this period, the patient is seen as an outpatient each week, for the removal of sutures, tightening of bolts, and later at 2 or 3 weekly intervals until the maxilla is firm enough for the removal of the external fixation. At about 8-10 weeks the intermaxillary fixation is released and then elastic bands are inserted between the arches to ensure that the osteotomy segments do not relapse. Extreme care is taken to prevent relapse and the elastic correction may well be continued for some time in order to control settling.

Fig. 10.6*a* shows the pre-operative views of a patient who is about to undergo a bimaxillary facial osteotomy for maxillary hypoplasia and

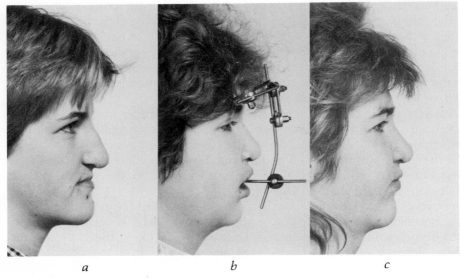

a   b   c

Fig. 10.6.

true mandibular prognathism. In *Fig.* 10.6*b* the osteotomy has been performed and the osteotomy is stabilized with cranio-maxillary fixation, and in *Fig.* 10.6*c* the fixation and splints have been removed.

Chapter 11

Genetic counselling

J. Osborne

This chapter will examine the complex aetiology of the cleft lip and palate deformity. Due to this complexity a parent of a cleft lip and palate baby wishing to know the chances of having another similarly affected child would be wise to consult a genetic counsellor.

There are many different causes giving rise to different patterns of disease, and the cleft lip or palate may be only one of the child's congenital abnormalities. Even so, the majority of children with cleft lip and palate do not have any other congenital abnormality.

Before any conclusion can be reached as to the aetiology in any single patient, a careful clinical examination must be performed both to confirm the type of defect and to look for other abnormalities. In addition a detailed family history is required, since there is an increased risk of affected children where even a third degree relative is affected.

Examination of both the index case and the relatives must be detailed, since associated defects may not be obvious. A cleft uvula of a relative will not be seen unless looked for and some defects, for example lip-pits, may be inconspicuous.

The information obtained from history and examination may allow the pattern of inheritance to be recognized as chromosomal, Mendelian, multifactorial or none of these. The commonest chromosomal causes are trisomy-13 and trisomy-18. These disorders are similar to Down's syndrome, in which there is no risk of cleft lip or palate, because in all three disorders there is a whole extra chromosome present in each cell in the body. This causes multiple congenital abnormalities, the pattern of which suggests the diagnosis. Confirmation is obtained by examination of the chromosomes. This type of disorder can happen to a mother at any age, but is more likely if the mother was elderly at the time of conception. Many of the children with trisomy-13 and trisomy-18 die in the first few weeks or months of life and they rarely need surgery to correct the cleft lip or palate.

There are a number of uncommon disorders which can be inherited in a Mendelian manner — the pattern of inheritance is dominant, recessive or X-linked. In dominant inheritance, an affected parent gives their child the same disorder. In recessive inheritance, both parents carry abnormal genes but are themselves normal adults. Their children have a high risk of disease. In X-linked inheritance, females with the abnormal gene are normal adults, but males with the abnormal gene have the disorder. Children whose cleft lip or palate has been inherited in one of these ways have other abnormalities which allow the disorder to be recognized and usually allow it to be named.

The majority of children with cleft lip or palate have inherited their disorder in a much less well understood way, called polygenic or multifactorial inheritance. In other words they have many factors operating which combine to cause the defect. There is no doubt that in some families a cleft palate alone is inherited as an isolated defect, while in other families a cleft lip is inherited which may be unilateral or bilateral and may or may not be associated with a cleft palate as well. In those families where a cleft palate is not associated with a cleft lip, there is no risk of any relative having a cleft lip. The risk of having an affected child depends on the number of people in the family already affected, and is increased if the affected member is a close relative. In addition, in families with cleft lips, the risk increases if there is also a cleft palate, and increases still further if the cleft lip is bilateral. If parents already have one child affected by a cleft lip with or without a cleft palate, then the risk to subsequent children is about one in twenty-five. If the affected child has a cleft palate alone the risk is about one in fifty for subsequent children. If two children have been affected the risk rises to one in ten for cleft lip with or without cleft palate, and one in twelve for cleft palate only, respectively. Children of an affected parent have a one in twenty-five or one in sixteen risk, respectively.

There are a number of other ways in which clefts can occur. Children with a cleft lip with or without a cleft palate who also have congenital heart disease are usually sporadic cases, and the risk to subsequent children is low. The cause of this is not known. Some children have the Robin anomaly (Pierre-Robin syndrome) in which slow development of the mandible (lower jaw) causes the tongue to prevent the fusion of the roof of the mouth, and a large, rather round cleft palate occurs. These babies usually have difficulty in breathing because the tongue gets in the way, and they may have to live in hospital for many weeks before going home. Subsequently the mandible usually catches up and the tongue is normally placed. The Robin anomaly is also sporadic in origin and the risk of further affected children is low.

It is well known that the children of epileptic mothers have babies with cleft lip or palate more often than other mothers. It is thought that some of the drugs used to treat epilepsy may cause the clefting, and phenytoin may do this most often, the risk being about one in fifty pregnancies. Unfortunately, the other drugs used to treat epilepsy are not yet known to be safer, and may cause more severe defects. It is usually considered unwise for a mother to take anticonvulsants during pregnancy unless it is really necessary. The most dangerous time to take them is during the first three months of pregnancy. Stopping these drugs must be done slowly, and is best done before attempting to become pregnant.

Recently, it has been shown that an ultrasound scan can be used to detect severe cleft lips. Cleft palates cannot yet be detected, and mild degrees of cleft lip with or without palate may be missed. An alternative method of antenatal diagnosis is by fetoscopy. This technique consists of introducing a sort of telescope into the uterus. This requires a small operation which may precipitate a miscarriage. The only purpose of such a test would be to offer the mother a therapeutic abortion if the baby were affected. Few doctors would feel that a cleft lip or palate alone justified abortion, which is usually performed for severe malformations.

Chapter 12

Family support

J.M. Smith

This chapter is devoted to the emotional, social and practical issues which face a family following the birth of a child with a cleft lip and palate.

Many trained people will be in contact with the parents soon after birth. It is important that each cleft lip and palate team has a clear policy to explain the problems to parents, both in hospital and later when the family returns home. Some areas in the United Kingdom can offer the benefits of willing advice given by the association of parents with previously treated cleft lip and palate children.

BIRTH

A cleft of the lip is an immediately visible handicap, and is distressing to the parents. It is important for maternity staff to be able to answer the more obvious questions about the problem and its management as soon as possible. Following this, specialists such as the plastic surgeon and orthodontist will see the cleft lip and palate child, preferably with the parents, to explain treatment management in more detail. To supplement this leaflets can be given, and in areas with a Cleft Lip and Palate Parents Association (CLAPA), parents of previously treated cleft children make themselves available to give encouragement and advice.

From birth to initial surgery is often a time of great stress. Many worries may develop, and everything that can be done by the cleft lip and palate team to allay these worries, will help the development of the relationship between the parents and their child.

On discharge from the hospital, the family's needs will be assessed. Their general medical practitioner and health visitor should be informed of the cleft problem. Where special difficulties exist, a social worker may be asked to help. These difficulties can include practical problems related to accommodation and finances, or problems of an emotional nature. The social worker and general medical practitioner are best placed to know of these particular problems, and how to help solve them. It is vital that trust and a good working relationship is developed between all those involved in the child's care. Much of the success of surgery and associated treatment rests on the quality of this relationship.

PRIMARY SURGERY

Babies usually have an operation to mend their lip at 3-6 months old. Where possible the mother should be with the child during the day in the ward. Some hospitals have facilities for mothers to 'live-in' close to the ward. Otherwise local boarding houses will provide a base for the mother who does not live in the vicinity of the hospital.

Parents should be given accurate information about the nature of the operation, and care following surgery. Good staff to parent communication can help prevent problems such as lack of interest in the baby, or rejection. Following surgery the baby will have his arms restrained to prevent thumbsucking, which could lead to break-down of the stitches. Spoon-feeding will be preferable following lip or palate surgery, to minimize disturbance of the surgical wound by vigorous sucking on a teat. The baby is likely to be in the ward for about two weeks.

A similar pattern will occur when the hard and soft palates are closed. A link between hospital and family at home can be maintained by the social worker.

CHILDHOOD

After the early lip and palate surgery, later corrective work may be necessary. When the child is old enough, it is important for plain explanations to be given about the surgery and stay in hospital. A visit to the ward, or play and story-telling, can be used to build up confidence and information about treatment. The parents may also need support because guilt about the deformity can prevent them from discussing the handicap with their child. Some families become so emotionally upset that they are unable to cope with the needs of their cleft child. Occasionally parents will protect their cleft child from normal children, thus intensifying the problem. In these circumstances professional help from the social worker and child guidance clinic may be necessary. The ultimate aim is to help parents understand the child and his needs.

EDUCATION

It is unlikely that a cleft child will need any special educational help, since it is unusual to have any other physical or mental handicaps. Parents and teachers should, however, be aware of the likelihood of fluctuating hearing loss and watch for signs at home, and in the classroom. The child may miss some schooling due to hospital admissions. It is important for parents to keep the school informed of such events. Teaching is now available in all hospitals, and teachers involved can liaise over appropriate studies.

ADOLESCENCE AND EARLY ADULTHOOD

It is important not to explain difficulty in behaviour as being the result of the physical deformity, rather than being due to normal adolescent problems. This deformity can be successfully treated by the combined efforts of many specialists. A team which communicates well with each other and with the parents and child will provide the best results.

Chapter 13

Feeding

I.S. Hathorn

The first few days, or even weeks, after the birth of a baby is a very anxious period for a mother striving to establish a satisfactory pattern of feeding. This can apply equally to cleft or non-cleft babies. For the mother who finds she has a baby with a cleft palate the problems will often seem greater. It needs to be emphasized that almost every baby with a cleft will learn to feed, since feeding is one of the most fundamental early needs comparable to the need to breathe.

Normal breast or bottle feeding takes place by sucking action where the lips surround the nipple or teat and the milk is pumped out by the thrusting action of the tongue and a negative pressure build-up within the baby's mouth. As will be seen in the chapter on classification of cleft lip and palate (*see* Chapter 3), the defects in lip and palate will vary. Those babies with a cleft of lip or soft palate only will have much less of a problem in feeding that those who have more complete clefts involving the hard palate and lip combined. In these latter babies there may be the additional problem of coordinating the reflex which allows steady breathing through the nose while continuing to suck. The most important single factor in helping the mother is the quality of reassurance which comes from having solved the problem many times before. A calm approach to these practical problems will help the anxious mother succeed in feeding. There are a number of ways in which the baby can be fed and a number of specialist aids to feeding. These are outlined below on an individual basis.

BREAST FEEDING

In the case of a mother who would like to establish breast feeding this should be concentrated upon within the first few days without the distraction of bottle feeding. For the cleft child with difficulty in generating the normal sucking pressures, it may not be possible to establish a flow of milk which is sustainable even with the aid of breast pumps. If this fails, the mother needs reassurance that this is not disastrous for her baby or that she herself has in some way failed.

BOTTLE FEEDING

Most babies with cleft of lip and palate will need to be bottle fed. Because of the poor ability to suck, help can be gained principally from opening up the hole in the teat so that a more effective flow of milk will take place. An adequate flow of milk from the bottle is, however, the most important means of aiding bottle feeding and the hole can be enlarged by using a red hot needle held in tweezers. It should be modified to suit the needs of the baby and it is usually best to use a standard teat in the first instance and, if there are problems, then specialist teats are now available which can be used to give further help. Some maternity units have found the large lambs teat works well. A recently available teat, the 'Nuk' teat, has a flat shape which has the advantage that it will straddle the cleft more effectively and it too benefits from changing the hole size. It seems that the best position for the hole is on the upper surface.

For some babies with a wide cleft of palate it is possible to fit a simple acrylic plate to cover the cleft defect and produce a normal arch form for the tongue to work against.

SPOON FEEDING

It is considered by most hospital staff involved in the care of cleft babies that considerable effort should be given to establishing a sucking routine. It is sometimes not possible and for these babies spoon feeding can be used. A most useful combination of spoon feeding is provided by the 'Rosti' bottle which consists of a plastic bottle with a large hole in the cap through which the milk can be expressed into a shallow gutter-like spoon. The 'Rosti' bottle is very useful for feeding babies just after operation when it is undesirable for the baby to suck against the freshly operated roof of the mouth.

TUBE FEEDING

This is used as a last resort usually only in premature babies which may have other medical problems. The baby will be under medical and nursing care during this period. As the baby gets stronger it will be gradually weaned onto spoon or bottle feeding.

Before a cleft baby is discharged from hospital a good feeding routine should be established. Individual feeding times for babies can be quite variable and it is important for mother and baby to reduce these times where possible.

Follow-up care on discharge from hospital is sometimes necessary for those babies who continue to have problems and it will serve to continue building up confidence and reinforcing the new feeding regime. It is fortunate that the need to feed is great since this will over-ride the temporary physical problem of the cleft.

Glossary

Accessory nerve: The eleventh cranial nerve (motor) supplying certain soft palate muscles, pharyngeal and laryngeal regions

Acrylic: The material from which dentures are made

Acrylic wafer: A surgical template to locate the bite at surgery

Active plate: A dental plate shaped to cause a change in the shape or relationship of parts of the upper alveolus

Adenoids: Lymphoid material within the naso-pharynx

Adenoidectomy: Surgical removal of adenoids

Aetiology: The cause of a disorder

Alveolus: Gum and bone containing teeth

Anaemia: A deficiency of red blood cells

Articulation: Dental: The functional relationship between two or more teeth. Speech: The enunciation of speech

Aspirate voice: Breathy; the use of excessive initial air flow preceding phonation

Audiometry: Measurement of the perception of sound

Bi-labials: Speech sounds produced at the lips, e. g. 'b', 'm'

Bronchi: Branches of the trachea in the lungs

Buccal sulcus: The furrow between the cheek and the teeth and gum

Cancellous bone: The soft interior of mature bone

Canines: Pointed teeth at the side of the incisor teeth

Cephalogram: A lateral skull X-ray film taken in a cephalostat (a device to hold the patient's head in a fixed position)

Chromosome: Threads of nucleoprotein carrying the hereditary characteristics of the individual

Concha: The cup of the external ear

Congenital: Actually or potentially present at birth

Connective tissue: A tissue which binds and supports the other elements of an organ

Crossbite: Upper teeth biting partly or completely inside lower teeth

Consonant cluster: A combination of two or more consonants, e.g. 'sp' or 'str'

Deciduous dentition: The first set of teeth acquired in infancy, which are shed and replaced by the permanent teeth

Differential growth: One body tissue growing faster than another and therefore changing relationships

Dental lamina: The layer of cells in the fetal mouth from which teeth will develop

Diagnostic therapy: A trial period of speech therapy to ascertain whether the over-riding problem has an anatomical basis or is learned behaviour

Ectoderm: Covering layer of cells in the fetus

Effusion: A pouring out of fluid

Endoderm: Lining layer of cells in the fetal body cavity or blood vessels

Epithelium: Covering layer of cells of the body or its cavities

Eustachian tube: The canal connecting the throat with the middle ear

Expressive speech: Communication using words

Extrinsic muscles: Originating or lying outside a part but acting on it

Facial nerve: The seventh cranial nerve (motor and sensory) controlling and coordinating muscles of facial expression

Fistula: An abnormal connection between two body cavities, e. g. between the mouth and nose, via the palate

Genioplasty: An operation to move the bony point of the chin forwards or backwards

Glossopharyngeal nerve: The ninth cranial nerve (sensory and motor) to tongue and pharynx — assists in swallowing

Glottalization: The substitution or co-articulation of a glottal stop for or with a consonant sound, e. g. 't', 's'

Glottal stop: A cough-like sound produced by the sudden release of a pulse of voiced or unvoiced air from the vocal folds

Hypernasality: Excess nasal tone heard on vowel sounds

Hypoglossal nerve: The twelfth cranial nerve supplying most of intrinsic and extrinsic muscles of the tongue

Hyponasality: Insufficient nasal tone (i.e. when nose blocked by a cold)

Image intensifier: Electrical — magnification of X-ray signals allowing lower doses of X-ray to produce clear images

Incisive foramen: Small openings in hard palate at the junction in the midline between the pre-maxilla and posterior palatal segments

Incisive papilla: Small nipple-shaped eminences of mucosa

Incisors: The four anterior teeth in each jaw

Index case: The first person in the family known to be affected

Intravenous infusion: The slow injection of a liquid into a vein

Intrinsic muscles: Situated within a part

Lip-pits: Congenital small indentations in the lips

Mandible: The lower jaw

Maxilla: The upper jaw

Maxillo-facial: Relating to the jaws and face

Mendelian: Patterns of inheritance discovered by Gregor Mendel who experimented by cross-breeding peas

Meninges: Three covering membranes of the brain and spinal cord

Meningitis: Inflammation of the membranes around the brain or spinal cord

Mesenchyme: Embryonic tissue giving rise to blood and to various types of connective tissue

Mucoperiosteum: A mucous surface immediately related to periosteum

Mucosa: Relating to mucous membrane

Mucous membrane: The membrane containing mucous glands and lining, for example the mouth or respiratory tract

Myofunctional therapy: Muscle-training therapy

Myotomes: The side and lower portions of primitive segments in the embryo

Myringotomy: Incision of the ear drum

Nasal cavity: Nose

Nasal escape: The audible or inaudible release of air down the nose during the production of a speech sound

Nasal pharyngoscopy: Examination of the pharynx using an endoscope passed through the nose

Nasal septum: The partition between left and right nasal passages

Naso-pharyngoscope: An instrument for viewing the nasal passages and pharynx

Naso-pharynx: The part of the throat above the soft palate

Obturator: An acrylic plate like a denture to close a hole in the palate

Occipital: Back of the head

Occlusion: The contacting relationship between the teeth of the upper and lower jaw

Oral cavity: Mouth

Oro-pharynx: The part of the pharynx at the back of the mouth

Orthopaedics: The realignment of the bony segments in cleft palate

Orthopantomogram: A composite X-ray of the teeth and jaws made by rotating the X-ray machine around the head to produce a flat picture of the entire mandible

Ossification: The process of laying down bone

Osteotome: A chisel-like instrument, sharpened on both sides

Osteotomy: The cutting of a bone

Otitis media: Inflammation of the middle ear

Otoscope: An instrument used to examine the external ear and ear drum

Overbite: The vertical overlap of the tips of upper teeth over lower teeth

Overjet: The horizontal overlap of upper teeth to lower teeth

Palatalization: Raising of the front of the tongue towards the hard palate appropriately as in 'sh' or inappropriately, e.g. for alveolar sounds when 's' becomes 'sh'

Palatal shelf: Left and right plates of palatal bone which develop to fuse in the mid-line to form the hard palate

Periosteum: The fibrous bone forming membrane investing the surfaces of bones

Pharyngeal plexus: A network of nerves situated on the constrictor muscles of the throat

Pharyngoplasty: An operation which changes the shape of the velo-pharyngeal isthmus

Pharynx: Throat — behind the nose (naso-pharynx), mouth (oro-pharynx) and tongue (hypo-pharynx)

Phonological: The functional behaviour of sounds for distinctive purposes

Plate (dental): An appliance worn in the mouth, usually made of acrylic

Premaxilla: Bone between the two parts of the upper jaw carrying the incisor teeth

Pre-medication: Sedative drug given before administering general anaesthetic

Procline: To incline forward

Prognathism: An abnormally projecting jaw

Pterygoid plate: Vertical bony plate(s) extending from the base of the skull behind the maxilla

Recurrent laryngeal nerve: A branch of the vagus nerve controlling laryngeal muscles and through them the vocal cord; sensory fibres below the vocal cord

Respiratory tract: The parts concerned with breathing, i.e. lungs, bronchi, trachea, larynx, pharynx, oral and nasal cavities

Resuture: To restitch

Retainer appliances: Following active orthodontics a retainer plate, usually made in acrylic, is fitted to hold the teeth in their new position

Retrocline: To incline backwards

Retro-gnathia: Receding jaw

Sensori-neural: A hearing loss associated with the inner rather than the middle ear

Settling: Changes in the dentition following surgery

Sinusitis: Inflammation within the sinuses

Sporadic: Occurring by chance

Submucous cleft: A cleft of the muscles of the soft palate with an intact covering of mucous membranes

Supernumerary: Of teeth; an extra tooth with an abnormal shape

Tinnitus: A ringing sound in the ear

Tonsillectomy: Surgical removal of the tonsils (lymph follicles enveloped in mucous membranes)

Trachea: Windpipe

Uterus: Womb

Uvula: The conical muscular body hanging from the free border of the soft palate

Vagus nerve: The tenth cranial nerve — sensory and motor nerve to the laryngeal muscles and some pharyngeal muscles, it regulates the contents of the body cavities

Vascular: Relating to the blood vessels

Velarization: The movement of the back of the tongue against the soft palate for some sounds, e.g. 'k', sometimes inappropriately, e.g. 't' realized as 'k'

Velopharyngeal competence: The ability of the velopharyngeal mechanism (comprising soft palate, lateral and posterior pharyngeal walls) to close completely when required during speech

Velum: Soft palate

Vestibule: The anterior compartment of the mouth

Vomerine bone: Bone forming lower and posterior part of nasal septum

Index